The
Chronic Disease
of
OBESITY

Other books written by Brian Scott Edwards, MD, FNLA

The Fen-Fen Diet Pill Program
The Tubby Theory from Topeka
The Tubby Traveler from Topeka

The
Chronic Disease
of
OBESITY

*How Sponge Syndrome Causes Repeated
Weight Gain*

Brian Scott Edwards, MD, FNLA

Board certified by American Board of Obesity Medicine

iUniverse

THE CHRONIC DISEASE OF OBESITY
HOW SPONGE SYNDROME CAUSES REPEATED WEIGHT GAIN

iUniverse books may be ordered through booksellers or by contacting:

iUniverse
1663 Liberty Drive
Bloomington, IN 47403
www.iuniverse.com
1-800-Authors (1-800-288-4677)

ISBN: 978-1-5320-6055-7 (sc)
ISBN: 978-1-5320-6056-4 (e)

Library of Congress Control Number: 2018912355

Print information available on the last page.

iUniverse rev. date: 10/25/2018

Dedicated to my wife, Virginia

The number of fat cells have the last word.

—Mark Edwards

Contents

Disclaimer

This book has a controversial viewpoint on maintaining weight loss. Please discuss changes in your diet, exercise, and medication with your physician. I do not know your personal medical history and can't advise specific changes for you as an individual. Diet medicines can be obtained only by a prescription from your physician, and two of them are DEA (Drug Enforcement Agency) controlled substances. Diet medications drugs should be taken for weight loss and then continued for the rest of your life to maintain weight loss by physician's prescription.

Foreword

I went to Dr. Brian Edwards as a friend on October 22, 2015. I was desperate because I was not getting better after working with my family physician and two rheumatologists. My legs were swollen despite being on two diuretics. I was taking allopurinol for the painful bumps on my wrists, which a biopsy revealed consisted of uric acid. My sugar was out of control and I could not lose weight.

Dr. Edwards advised some changes. He wanted me to switch to an Atkins-type diet immediately, slowly decrease insulin, and slowly increase Invokana. He also told me to stop the diuretics, start colchicine, start metformin up to 2,000 mg a day, and get a sleep apnea test. Later when my rheumatologist wanted to put me on prednisone, Dr. Edwards said absolutely not to do it and my family physician agreed.

By November 28, 2015, I was totally off insulin. On January 15, 2016, I was on Invokana 300 mg, metformin 2,000 mg, and no insulin. My Hgb A1c had dropped from 7.6 to 6.5 with a weight of 318 pounds. Dr. Edwards asked my family physician to start Victoza and slowly increase the dose. On February 24, 2016, I was on a full diabetic dose of Victoza, 1.8 mg. My results were miraculous.

October 22, 2015
First weigh-in at Dr. Edwards's home with a Valhalla total body composition scale:
Weight 348 pounds
Body fat 52.9%
Muscle mass 32.2 pounds
Body water 38.2%
BMI 57.8

March 8, 2016
I hit a low weight of 308.8, and I had lost forty pounds.

June 25, 2016
Dr. Edwards started me on Contrave to help stop my cravings and to continue or at least maintain weight loss.
Weight 319.4 pounds
Body fat 51%
Muscle mass 30.9 pounds
Body water 38.7%
BMI 52.8

November 12, 2016
My last total body weight composition at Dr. Edwards's free clinic:
Weight 309.6 pounds
Body fat 51%
Body water 38.9%
Muscle mass 30.6 pounds
Fasting glucose around this time was usually 142.

I know these numbers because Dr. Edwards set up a spreadsheet on Google Docs for me. He had me type in my weight and fasting glucose every day as he followed along on his computer.

I am grateful to Dr. Edwards for his treatment of me for one year.

Anonymous

Preface

Wake-up call: So many things in the ACC/AHA guidelines are wrong, and guidelines usually set out only minimum requirements. For example, the guidelines are still using LDLc levels instead of LDL particle counts (LDLp). Also, the National Lipid Association (LPA) has progressed to using non-HDL cholesterol (non-HDLc) goals, which I proposed in *The Tubby Theory from Topeka* back in 2010.[5] Non-HDLc includes all cholesterol except the HDLc. I called this the Tubby Factor.[32]

Other mistakes in the guidelines:

1. Advising the use of very expensive PCSK9 IV drugs instead of low-dose, inexpensive, generic triple therapy to get to the very lowest LDLp. Triple therapy is the lowest dose of statin, ezetimibe, and only 1,000 mg of Endur-Acin (niacin). I found Endur-Acin to be effective with fewer side effects than brand name niacin.
2. Taking inexpensive niacin off the alternative drug list to statins. They made this decision based on data that turned out to insignificant after further analysis.[33]
3. Not understanding the sponge theory as a reason for regaining weight, and advising diet and exercise for maintaining weight loss despite the failure of this approach in the Look AHEAD trial.
4. Believing that the obese can "outrun their fork."
5. Thinking that a calorie is a calorie.
6. Believing that the reduced obese can maintain their weight with exercise.

I've reviewed the two best diet books of 2016: *Always Hungry* by David Ludwig and *The Change Your Biology Diet* by Louis J. Aronne. These are good books that reflect the move away from low-fat diets. These two books also reflect the general opinion that Atkins is too restrictive on carbohydrates and thus cannot be continued for more than six to ten months.

Both books put forth diets allowing more carbohydrates that have low glycemic indexes. "This will slowly reprogram your fat cells," Dr. Ludwig claims.[1] My problem with this is that I don't believe it affects the low leptin levels.

Dr. Aronne goes one step further by claiming that ten minutes twice a week of high-intensity exercise will make the difference, as long as you do the exercise until you reach muscle failure.[2] My problem with this idea is that it might lead to injuries, especially in the elderly. Instead, I suggest that people do three sets of twenty-five repetitions with low weights four days a week. When combined with eating 2.4 grams of protein/kg lean body weight, this preserves muscle mass with weight loss. This is difficult, but probably easier than fewer repetitions with heavier weights. Start with one set the first week, and then increase another two sets over two weeks. You will know the correct weight for you, because the last three repetitions should burn your muscles.

After I passed the American Board of Obesity Medicine exam in December 2015, I was astonished to realize that my professors were still selling the old diet and exercise routine. We know from the failed ten-year Look AHEAD trial[3] that diet and exercise don't work over the long term. At obesity meetings, Dr. Aronne has suggested that multiple diet medications are the answer for some people.

In my preparation for the Obesity Boards, I went to several conferences. The physicians with the most clinical experience taught that the guidelines are wrong, because you cannot outrun your fork. The guidelines tell the reduced obese that to maintain their weight loss, they simply need to walk an hour a day and maintain a 1,200–1,500-calorie diet. This is what people do who have maintained weight loss in the National Weight Control Registry (NWCR).

The American Board of Obesity Medicine (ABOM) lecturers pointed to the Minnesota Starvation Experiment, as documented in Todd Tucker's book, *The Great Starvation Experiment: Ancel Keys and the Men Who Starved for Science*.[4] At the end of World War II, Dr. Keys put thirty-two conscientious objectors on a starvation diet and exercised them for twenty-four weeks. They were on 1,550 calories a day and walked an hour a day. The men were so miserable that many of them began eating garbage, which got them kicked out of the program in shame.

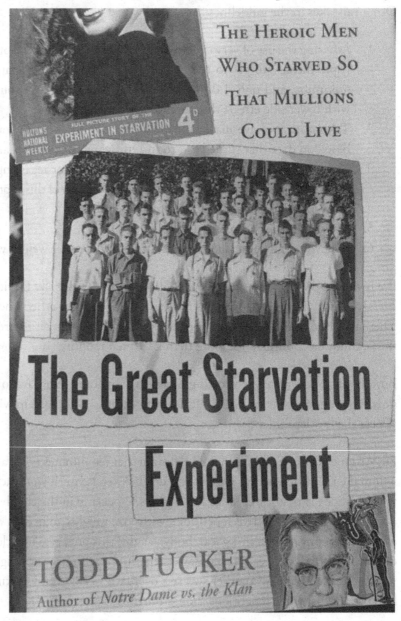

The guidelines expect our reduced obese patients to follow the same starvation level of calories and exercise for the rest of their lives just to maintain their weight loss. Ten thousand people in the NWCR have said they are able to do it.

This starvation diet was also given to prisoners of war during World War II in Japan: 1.25 cup of white rice (300 calories) for three meals per day. They also got 400 cc of soup, which was probably between 200 and 400 calories.

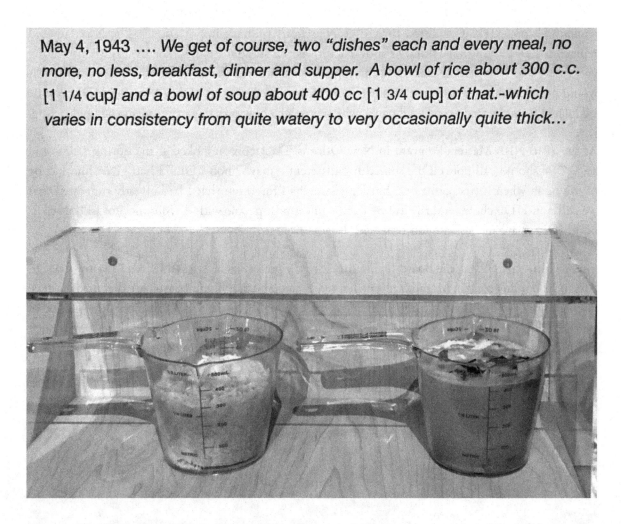

May 4, 1943 .... *We get of course, two "dishes" each and every meal, no more, no less, breakfast, dinner and supper. A bowl of rice about 300 c.c. [1 1/4 cup] and a bowl of soup about 400 cc [1 3/4 cup] of that.-which varies in consistency from quite watery to very occasionally quite thick...*

Source: World War II exhibit at Kansas State University. Please go to my blog, *The Tubby Traveler from Topeka*, to see a photo of the exhibit and the food given to the prisoners.

This idea of staying on a starvation diet just to maintain weight loss has not truly been embraced by the nutrition obesity industry, because they feel it is too dark. I faced a similar situation after I passed the Boards of the National Lipidology Association (NLA) in 2007. Tim Russert had died, and no lipidologist had spoken up and claimed that Russert had not been treated correctly according to guidelines. That's why I wrote *The Tubby Theory from Topeka*.[5]

I coined the term *Tubby Factor* to replace the complicated term *non-HDL cholesterol (non-HDLc)*. Mr. Russert's non-HDLc was not at goal, and I suspect that his physician had no idea what that goal should have been. Certainly none of the cardiologists on TV ever mentioned it.

I also proposed a way to reduce the 100,000 sudden coronary deaths every year by recommending that a CAC (CT of heart) and/or CIMT (carotid intimal wall thickening ultrasound) be done on anyone who has at least one risk factor.

Interestingly, my ideas, which originated with my professors at the NLA, were validated by the *Journal of Clinical Lipidology* in 2015: "Although both non-HDL-C and LDL-C are termed atherogenic cholesterol, non-HDL-C is listed first to emphasize its primary importance."[6] The NLA advised replacing LDLc with non-HDLc (Tubby Factor) as the standard biomarker to use when treating patients. I said in my book that LDLp or apoB should become the standard, but I knew the NLA would never reach consensus on that since most of the trial data used LDLc. Also non-HDLc can be calculated from the traditional lipid panel, which is much cheaper than getting advanced lipid testing.

At the 2016 NLA Masters Program in New Orleans, Dr. Jacobson looked at me during a class and said, "We should call non-HDLc something different—maybe non-LDL." I had given him a copy of my book when it first came out, but I guess he had forgotten that I had already suggested that we call non-HDL cholesterol the Tubby Factor since most people with discordance (of LDLc versus non-HDLc) have metabolic syndrome with large waists.

Once again, after passing the Boards in obesity, I see my professors hedging their bets. I know that Dr. Aronne is holding back in his medication chapter, because he taught me how to use diet medications. He uses multiple diet medications in some patients, though with no trials to support the success of that strategy except with Contrave (naloxone/buspirone) and Qsymia (phentermine/topiramate). Many physicians also are giving their diabetes type 2 patients metformin, Invokana, and lower-dose liraglutide. To date, there have been no trials on patients who take five drugs, just the experience of many diabetic patients who are also being treated for obesity.

Introduction

Most people can't maintain their weight loss. I maintained my eighty-pound weight loss after giving up on extreme exercise and switching to an Atkins ad libitum (eating until full) diet, but more importantly by taking multiple diet medications.

Summary of my major weight loss with medications:

- Invokana 300 mg 3-4-14 (262 lb.) to 6-24-15 (244 lb.)
- Qsymia 6-24-15 (244 lb) to 11-9-16 (213.4 lb)
- Belviq 10 mg BID 11-15-16 (212.4 lb.) to 3-1-17 (212.4 lb.)
- Liraglutide to 3.0 mg (maximum dose for dieting) on 3-1-17 (212.4 lb. on Hawaii scale) to (200.8 lb. on Topeka scale).

It was also very important to stop insulin and Actos, since these two drugs cause weight gain.

These multiple diet medications have helped me maintain my weight loss from 280 pounds in February 2006 to 200 pounds twelve years later. Atkins was essential, because I *was never hungry*. This is the type of diet I could eat for the rest of my life. I didn't really lose weight on Atkins; I mostly stopped gaining weight even though I decreased my daily exercise from two hours to walking twenty to forty minutes. I documented my weight maintenance of 246 pounds during 2011 as I went on cruises and traveling around the world in my book *The Tubby Traveler from Topeka*.[7]

I lost significant weight when I added Invokana (canagliflozin), which is indicated for diabetes. I used it to replace insulin in my type 2 diabetes mellitus. Invokana causes approximately 200 calories of glucose to be lost in the urine each day. My last Hgb. A1c was 6.7 on 6-6-17.

Not everyone will lose weight with Invokana. I was also taking Victoza 1.8 mg at the time. I later started Qsymia and after sixteen months I replaced it with Belviq. The diet medicines circumvented the sponge syndrome, which is caused by the high number of fat cells retained from my peak weight of 280 pounds.

I maintained a thirty-pound weight loss from January 2011 with Atkins ad libitum and twenty to forty minutes walking. From June 24, 2015, I lost another forty-four pounds by adding Qsymia and later switching to Belviq and increasing my liraglutide dose to 3.0 mg a day.

This is the message my book is going to convey. It's all about finding a diet you can stay on for life and the medication you will need as weight regain occurs because of the sponge syndrome.

Abbreviations

Obesity science

MiRNA: micro (small noncoding) RNA

NPY/AgRP neurons: activated by ghrelin (ghrelin stimulates NPY release; AgRP release increases orexigenic pathway)

MSH: melanocyte stimulating hormone

VMH: ventromedial hypothalamus

POMC: proopiomelanocortin

LCHF: low carbohydrate, high fat

Medical imaging

CIMT: carotid intimal wall thickening (an ultrasound test)

CAC: coronary artery calcium (measured on a CT scan of heart)

Blood tests

LDL: low density lipoprotein

LDLc: specifically LDL cholesterol (usually is calculated)

LDLp: specifically LDL particle number done by NMR (nuclear magnetic resonance)

ApoB: particle count done usually by immune assay

HDL: high density lipoprotein

non-HDLc: all the cholesterol without the HDLc, including remnants

Associations

NLA: National Lipid Association

FNLA: Fellow of National Lipid Association

OMA: Obesity Medical Association

TOS: The Obesity Society

Diabetes

IR: insulin resistance

Cholesterol-lowering drugs

PCSK-9: proprotein convertase subtilisin/kexin (an enzyme encoded by the PCSK-9 gene)

PCSK-9 inhibitor: a new type of drug (such as alirocumab) that binds the protein and, paradoxically, lowers cholesterol. PCSK-9 destroys the liver's PCSK-9 receptor. Normally the PCSK-9 receptor clears cholesterol to be destroyed and recycled; hence my use of the word *paradoxical*. See guidelines.[8]

My Chronic Obesity Weight Record

September 1960—115 lb.
Second grade, age 9

August 31, 1964—150 lb.
5 feet 5 inches, age 12
BMI 25, 95th percentile on growth chart

September 19, 1965—175 lb.
5 feet 8.5 inches, age 13
BMI 26, 95th percentile on growth chart

October 30, 1967—185 lb.
5 feet 9 inches, age 15
Started Weight Watchers diet

April 1968—160 lb.
5 feet 10 inches, age 16
70th percentile on growth chart

June 30, 1969—166 lb.
Waist 33.5 inches

June 17, 1970—173 lb.
5 feet 11 inches, age 19
BMI 24, waist 35 inches

July 2, 1970—164 lb.
Waist 34 inches
Ran mile in 5 minutes, 20 seconds

December 5, 1972—200 lb.

January 17, 1973—180 lb.

January 10, 1974—194 lb.
Waist 38.25 inches

1988

In my first big weight loss, I went from 245 pounds to 208 pounds while working at my first medical practice in Clermont, Florida. I attended Overeaters Anonymous meetings, went to Nautilus and lifted weights three times a week, and jogged daily while on 1,000 calories. I stayed at this weight for a few months, but the deprivation was too much, and I quickly went back up to 220 pounds.

October 1995—272 lb.
Waist 49 inches.
I could bench press 340 pounds free weight. I went on Fastin and Pondimin.

1996—220 lb.
Waist 42 inches, age 45

1998—240 lb.
Age 47

February 2006—280 lb.

November 2006—200 lb.

December 2010—250 lb.

March 1, 2014—265 lb.
I started Invokana and stopped insulin. My glucose immediately improved, dropping below 150. I went down to 239.5 lb. without changing my diet or exercise.

June 25, 2015—244.8 lb.
Waist 43 inches

Weighed in at Stormont Vail Obesity Clinic, started Qsymia, and lost 21 lb.

November 15, 2016—212.4 lb.
Switched to Belviq 10 mg BID. I had to stop Qsymia because of fast heart rate. I did not lose more weight with Belviq, but I achieved my goal of maintaining my weight loss.

March 1, 2017—212.4 lb.
I changed my 1.8 mg diabetic dose of Victoza (liraglutide) to a 3 mg diet dose of Saxenda (liraglutide) on the first day of my Hawaii vacation, because I was incorrectly told that I had to lose another 5 percent to be allowed to stay on the diet drugs.

May 31, 2017—203 lb.
I went back to the 1.8 mg diabetic dose of Victoza (liraglutide).

July 27, 2017—199 lb.

December 10, 2017—214.4 lb.
Increased Victoza from 1.8 to Saxenda dose of 3 mg (diet dose for liraglutide)

January 5, 2018—203.2 lb.
Decreased Victoza to 1.8 mg (diabetic dose)

My Chronic Obesity Photos

I always thought I was a chubby child. I pulled up some photos to document it.

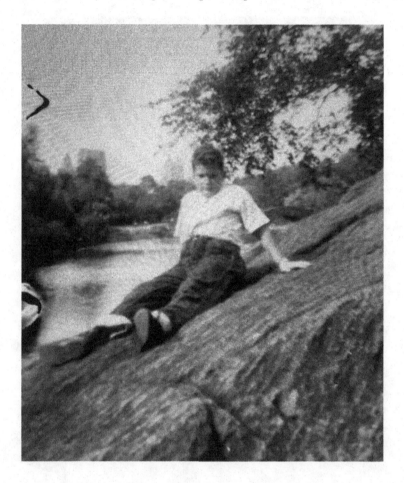

July 1958
Age 7 years, 7 months
Summer in Central Park, New York City. I was called *husky* size at this age.

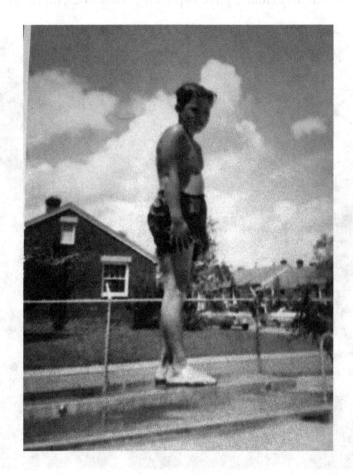

August 1960
Age 9 years, 8 months
A big kid for my age, I thought I was overweight. I ate a tremendous amount and was very active. I finished second grade.

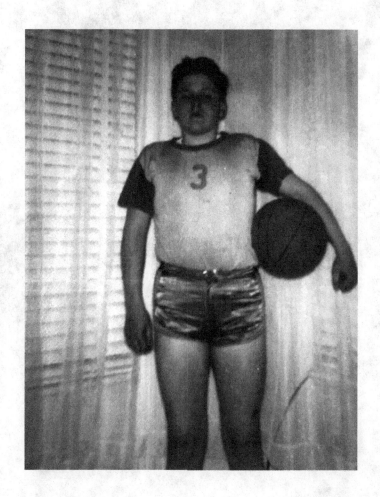

October 1963
Age 12 years, 10 months
Sixth grade at Public School 89 in Brooklyn, New York

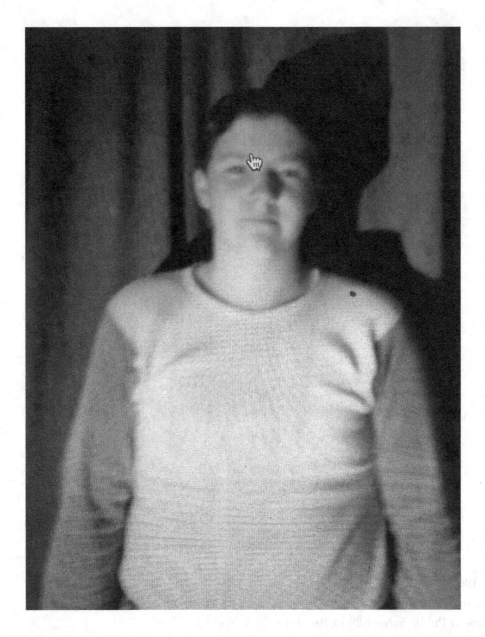

April 1965
Age 14 years, 4 months
Seventh grade at Andreas Hudde High School on school basketball team. I went on the Weight Watchers diet during high school.

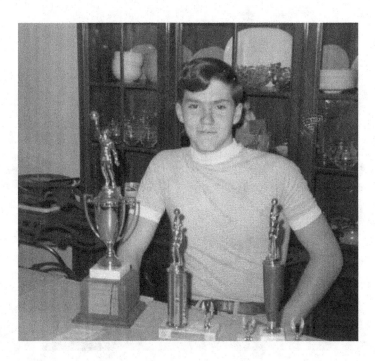

April 1968
Age 17 years, 4 months
At 5 feet 10 inches and 160 pounds, I'm a junior at Stuyvesant High School in Manhattan, in New York City. To get to this weight, I had been on Weight Watchers.

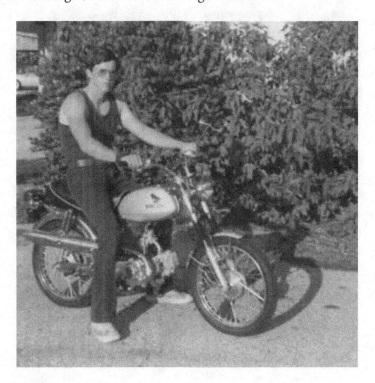

July 1970
Age 19 years, 7 months
After my first year at Brooklyn College

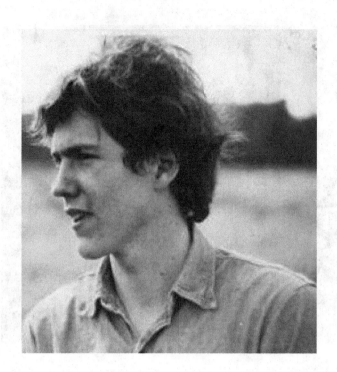

August 1972
Age 21 years, 8 months
Taken in Richmond Park, England

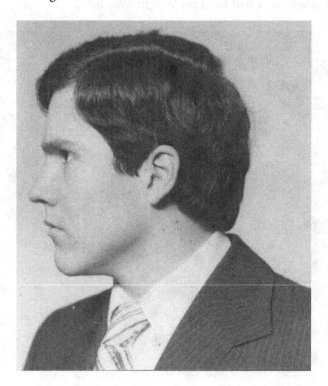

June 1977
Age 26 years, 6 months
I graduated from medical school.

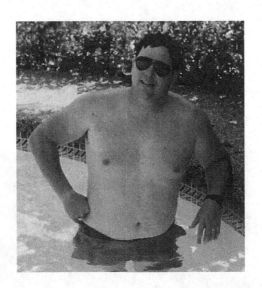

July 1988
Age 37, 245 pounds

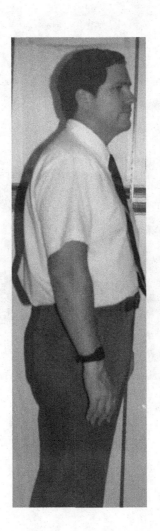

September 1989
Age 38, 208 pounds

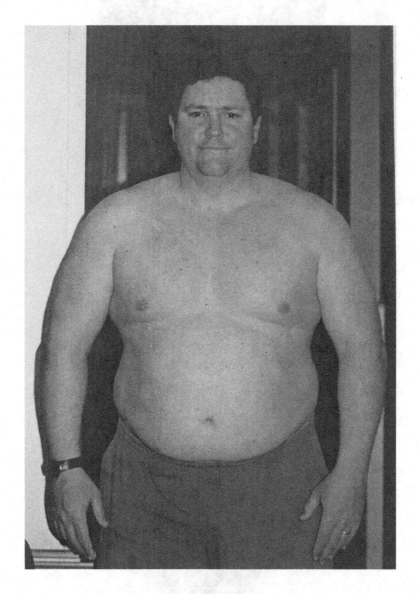

October 1995
Age 44, 272 pounds, waist 49 inches

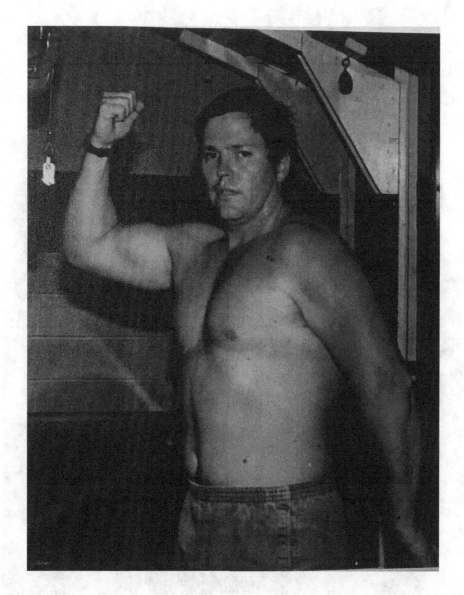

November 1996
Age 45, 220 pounds, waist 42 inches

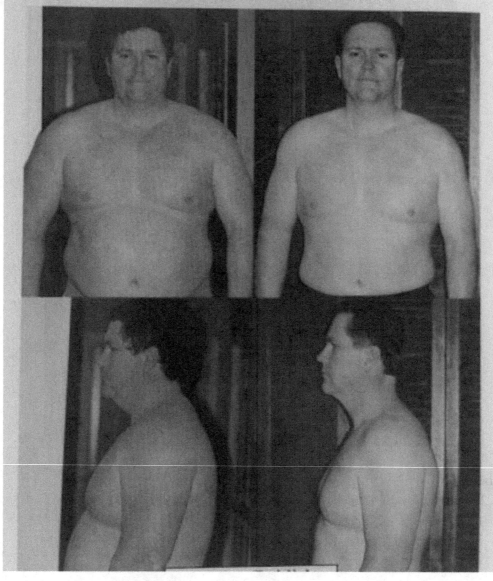

December 1996

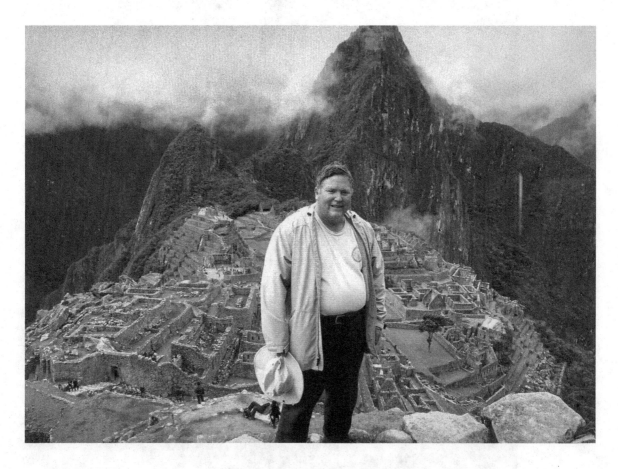

December 2005
Age 54, 280 pounds
In March 2006, I started *The 3-Hour Diet* by Jorge Cruise.

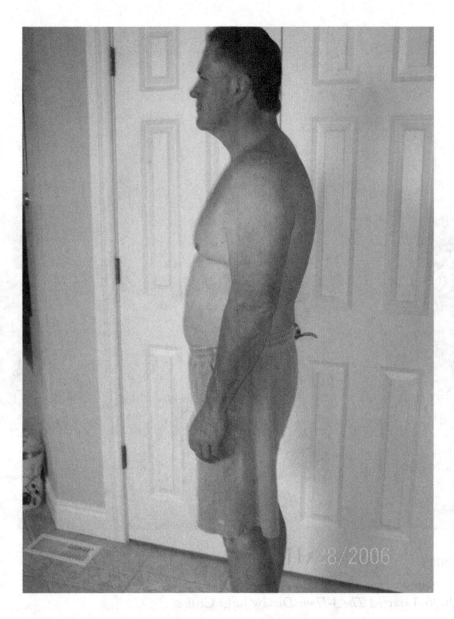

November 28, 2006
Age 55, 200 pounds

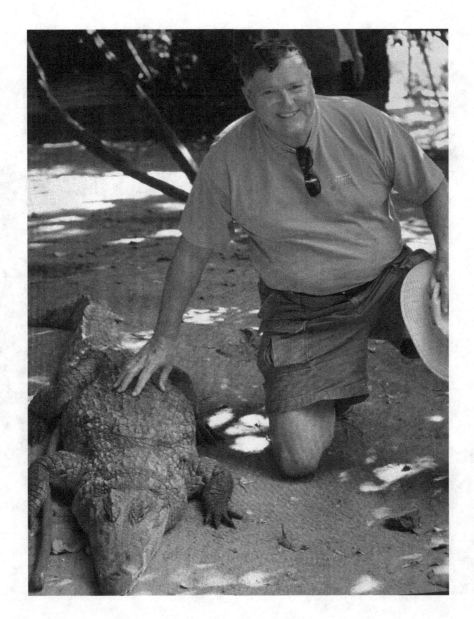

November 27, 2010
Age 58, 250 pounds

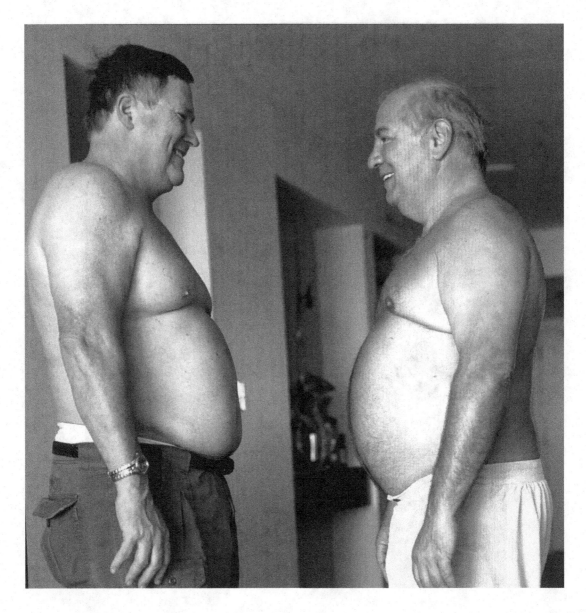

February 24, 2011
Age 59. I had been on the Atkins diet for a month without losing weight.

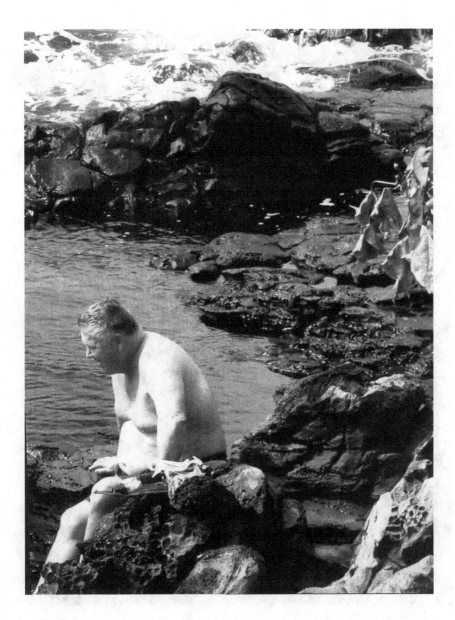

January 2014
Age 63, 260 pounds
I started Invokana and stopped insulin in March 2014. My glucose immediately improved, dropping below 150.

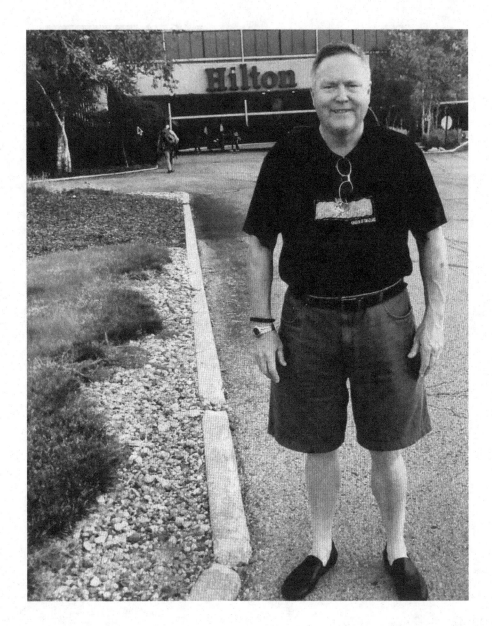

August 2014
Age 63, 239.5 pounds. No change in diet or exercise.

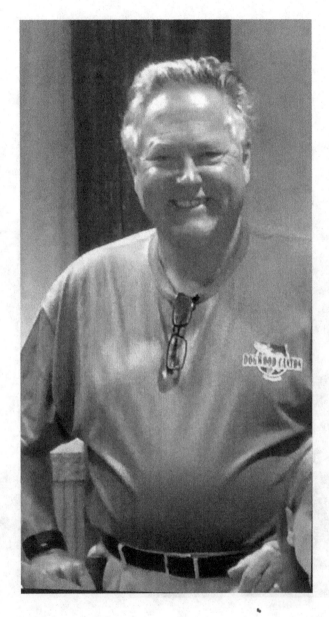

June 16, 2015
244.8 pounds, waist 43 inches
Weigh-in at Stormont Vail Obesity Clinic. I started Qsymia on June 24, 2015.

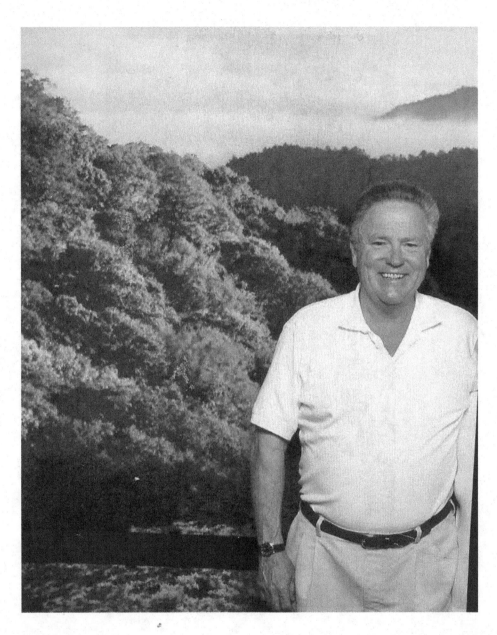

November 7, 2016
213.6 pounds. I switched to Belviq on November 15, 2016.

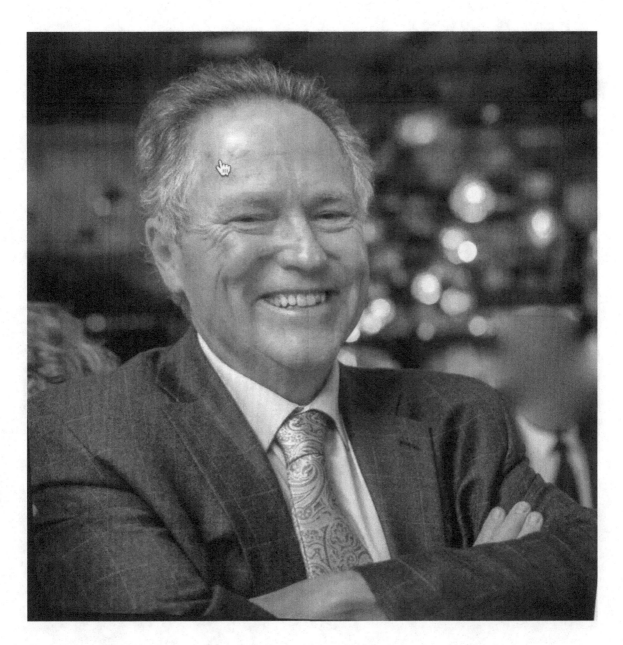

May 12, 2017
Age 65, 203.6 pounds
Wedding in Philadelphia

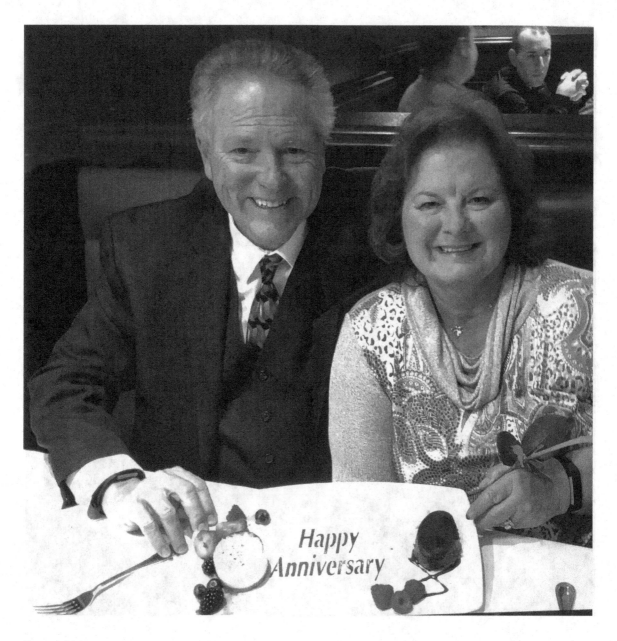

December 13, 2017
208.4 pounds
I'm having a great meal at the Capital Grill at the Plaza in Kansas City.

PART 1

Chronic Obesity

CHAPTER 1

How to Maintain Weight Loss

To maintain your weight loss, *you must stay on your reduced-calorie diet for life,* especially when you hit your plateau after six to nine months. That could be the end of this book. It is dark news.

The National Weight Control Registry (NWCR)[31] includes ten thousand people who have maintained their weight loss longer than five years. They stay on low-calorie diets ranging from 1,200 to 1,500 calories and walk an hour each day.

That's what works, so do it. The guidelines say it's all about having enough willpower to maintain your lifestyle. I don't understand why the guidelines discount the chemical pathways between gut, fat, and brain that cause weight regain when the body thinks it's starving. Leptin, insulin, and ghrelin are the big three.

The good news is that diet medications can help control your hunger when you hit your plateau and the sponge syndrome kicks in. However, the media and most doctors have not embraced this good news yet.

These are good books for losing weight:

- *The New Atkins for a New You,* by Eric C. Westman, Stephen D. Phinney, and Jeff S. Volek (2010)
- *Always Hungry?* by David Ludwig (2016)
- *The Change Your Biology Diet,* by Louis J. Aronne (2016)
- *The South Beach Diet,* by Arthur Agatston (2003)
- *The Diet Fix: Why Diets Fail and How to Make Yours Work,* by Yoni Freedhoff (2014)
- *Dr. Cohen's New Hippocratic Diet Guide,* by Irving A. Cohen (2008)

The problem is reading them and following them. None of them include supporting data. My book documents my eighty-pound weight loss maintained over eleven years, in a case study of one person. I ate Atkins ad libitum (until I was full) and was not hungry, while walking twenty to forty minutes each day. I also drank alcohol. Diet medications were the key to my success. In this book, I document my personal history of maintaining weight loss, from 280 pounds in March 2006 to 200 pounds in June 2017.

First: Keep it simple.

Keeping diaries for the rest of your life is not simple. Counting calories is not simple. I suspect the reduced obese who read this book have used diaries and calorie counting with short-term effectiveness.

The books mentioned above are various versions of the low-carbohydrate, high-fat diet (LCHF). They usually include "phases," which are too complicated for most patients. I truly doubt they make a difference in the long run for 90 percent of the reduced obese who are trying to maintain their weight loss. The phases are an attempt by the authors to get back to a less-restrictive diet for life. If that means more calories, the reduced obese will gain weight. All the books listed above include recipes, none of which I have ever used.

If you have successfully used one or more of these books as guides, I congratulate and admire you. Actually half of the people in NWCR have maintained their weight loss completely on their own. The people with this amazing willpower are the people scientists want in their trials. It appears that all weight loss diets or surgeries have "waterfall" results,[9] which means there a wide range of weight-loss results in both the tested group and the control group.

The Look AHEAD trial[10] was the biggest scientific effort to prove that diet and exercise will work over the long run to lower cardiovascular events. Why did it fail? Probably because the people in the control group were just as mentally and psychologically capable of doing it on their own in the long run. The waterfall results were very similar in both groups. After four years, there was only a 3.6 percent difference in weight loss between the control and treatment groups. (For more about waterfall results with diet and surgery trials, go to my blog.[9])

In the practice of clinical obesity, we don't get to choose our patients. Our patients want a magical pill that makes them lose weight, doesn't cost much, and has no side effects. Unfortunately they don't want to continue diet medications after they lose their weight, because they consider taking pills to be a crutch or too expensive.

Gastric bypass surgery is now seen as a magical procedure for many people. At one of my obesity conferences, a slide showed that 30 percent of bariatric surgery patients gain their weight back within ten years. A recent article showed that 20 percent of bariatric patients are on pain medications after several years.[11]

I weighed 280 pounds in March 2006 and lost eighty pounds in time for my wedding in June 2007. I did it the old-fashioned way, by counting calories and exercising one to two hours a day. (See *The Three Hour Diet* by Jorge Cruise.[12]) I was exhausted by the discipline and always hungry despite five meals a day. I decided to eat more fruit and increase my exercise to two hours and thirty minutes a day, but I gained a pound and a half a month until I had a regain of fifty pounds by 2011.

My big mistake was that instead of eating fruit for my midmorning and midafternoon snacks, I should have had a minimum of 10 grams of protein for each snack. I recommend these protein drinks:

- Protein Premier—30 grams of protein at 160 calories (3 grams of fat)
- Atkins shakes—15 grams of protein at 160 calories (9 grams of fat)
- EAS MYO—42 grams of protein at 300 calories (7 grams of fat) for intense weight lifters
- Premier Protein's Clear Protein Drink—20 grams of protein at 90 calories (no sugar). I add this to Powerade Zero Fruit Punch to cut the sweetness.[30]

Now that I am back down to 200 pounds, I plan to follow a protein diet of 150 grams a day and weight lifting (three sets of twenty-five repetitions) at least four times a week. Elderly men develop a condition called *sarcopenia*, which is loss of muscle mass, mostly in the legs. I try to lift weights every day, alternating upper body on even-numbered days and lower body on odd-numbered days, which does increase my appetite. I feel full but my cravings for certain foods continue, although a cup of caffeinated coffee in the afternoon helps. Certainly the diet medications prevent my hunger but not always the craving that may come with the boredom of a restrictive diet.

If you can keep carbs down to six days a week and not binge on them, the Atkins diet might still work for you. If I bring ice cream or a whole pizza into my house, I can't limit my portions. If I don't eat high protein (30 grams or more) at breakfast, lunch, and dinner, I get very hungry between meals. When I do get hungry between meals, I eat a snack that has at least 10 grams of protein. Even with the high-protein diet, the more I exercise, the hungrier I get.

I've found that diet medications clearly allow me to eat less on the same Atkins diet and exercise while still losing weight. Diet medications have also helped me not regain on the same diet and exercise without increased hunger.

In 2011, at the obesity teaching courses from the Obesity Society, in Orlando, Florida, I learned about leptin, the reduced obese state, and the billions of fat cells that remain in my body despite my eighty-pound weight loss.[28]

I was writing my book *The Tubby Traveler from Topeka*[7] and subsequently elucidated the sponge syndrome theory in 2011 as a result of the teaching of Dr. Rudolph L. Leibel[12] at the obesity conference. Weight loss from diet, exercise, and bariatric surgery causes billions of fat cells to shrink *but not to disappear,* and they continue to produce less leptin. Patients gain fat even at low calorie levels and high exercise levels because the body thinks it's starving. Neither diet, exercise, nor bariatric surgery reduces the *number* of fat cells—they only *shrink* them with weight loss. Liposuction removes fat cells, but then the body replaces them in different locations.

"After *The Biggest Loser*, Their Bodies Fought to Regain Weight," by Gina Kolata, has recently validated my sponge theory.[13] It's not the amount of lean muscle loss that causes the weight regain, but the amount of fat lost with the resultant low level of leptin in the remaining fat cells. The best way to prevent weight regain in the reduced obese is to address this low leptin level with multiple diet medications.

In addition to diet medications, to *maintain weight loss*, the patient has to

- find a restrictive diet that they can maintain for the rest of their life. It must be low in calories: 1,000–2,000 per day.
- weigh themselves every day and get right back on the strict diet at a three-pound gain.
- walk twenty minutes a day for health—not for weight loss.
- expect weight loss for only six to nine months.
- at plateau, not expect to break through with lower calories, more exercise, or even diet medications. Diet medications help you lose weight, but they should be continued for life to maintain weight loss with less hunger, allowing you to tolerate lower calories.

I would advise that after hitting the plateau with a diet that has worked for you in the past, you should stop counting calories and switch to an Atkins-type diet that is LCHF (low carbohydrate, high fat).

- Just don't eat carbohydrates.
- LCHF (Atkins) is ad libitum, meaning that you eat until you're full.
- You avoid hunger because of high protein and nutritional ketosis; thus you are satisfied with 500 fewer calories. The challenge is to stop eating when you're full.
- LCHF (Atkins) tastes good because of high fat.

At the plateau, the goal is simply to feel satisfied with the restrictive diet and not gain weight. If there is significant weight regain, it's time to begin taking diet medications or taking more of them.

The LCHF diet and diet medications should be continued for the rest of your life. *If you are not prepared to take diet medications for the rest of your life, you probably should not bother to start.* This is the treatment for the chronic disease of obesity.

If you do better with another diet and can stay on it for life, then by all means use what works, especially if you are not diabetic type 2 or pre-diabetic and don't have the metabolic syndrome. The LCHF diet is especially good for insulin-resistant patients.

Second: Discuss the diet medications below with your physician.

Contrave and Qsymia are combination medications that are "on label." However, it's easy to go "off-label" with diet medications as your physician individualizes your treatment. Going off-label means using medications to treat disorders not listed under FDA indications in the *Physicians' Desk Reference* (PDR).

The FDA anti-obesity medication indications are (1) a BMI greater than or equal to 30 kg/m2, or (2) a BMI greater than or equal to 27 kg/m2 with presence of diabetes mellitus, hypertension, and dyslipidemia.

In Kansas, the Stormont Obesity Clinic told me that I had to lose 5 percent of my weight to be allowed to take the diet medication for the rest of my life. For the reduced obese at plateau, this may not be feasible. They need the diet medications not only to lose more weight, but to maintain their weight. If you're worried that you cannot lose another 5 percent of weight after already hitting the plateau, start a high-protein diet with weight lifting. When you gain five to ten pounds of muscle, it may be possible to lose another 5 percent on the new diet pill. Ideally you can keep the muscle gain by continuing high protein (2.4 g/kg) and high reps with low weight resistance training four days a week.

I believe the federal guidelines simply want to see clinical improvement, rather than necessarily a 5 percent weight loss. If your osteoarthritis pain declines, that's a clinical improvement.

If you've tolerated a diet medication for twelve weeks and had some intermittent benefit, as I did with liraglutide (Victoza), don't give up on it. Adding Qsymia to the Victoza made a tremendous difference to my program. I was on six diet medications, but I switched from Qsymia to Belviq and I'm now on caffeine (coffee) and five medications: metformin, Invokana, Victoza, Qsymia (phentermine/topiramate), and Belviq (Locaserin).

I am also on an ad libitum Atkins diet, and I usually have a serum nutritional ketosis with ketone level greater than 0.5. I call my diet the *bon vivant diet* because I go on cruises and drink alcohol daily. I walk only one or two miles a day, and I recently started weight lifting.

It's easy to be "off-label" on diet medications. I went to a Saxenda presentation recently and was surprised to learn that I'm supposed to increase the dose every week up to the maximum. If a patient can't tolerate the maximum dose, they have to give up on the drug. They can't go back to the lower dose without side effects, even though they've had an effective weight loss of 5 percent. However, if the patient tolerates the high dose and loses weight, they can cut the Saxenda to a lower dose if they wish.

Victoza and Saxenda are exactly the same drug (liraglutide). Saxenda, which comes in higher doses, has a 40 percent side-effect report. Despite this high rate of side effects, most people are able to tough through the nausea and stay on the drug. I had abdominal pain on Victoza, so I backed off for a while and returned to it more slowly. A physician has to be allowed to treat patients on an individual basis.

Your physician might ask you to sign a document acknowledging that you're taking a drug off-label for something not indicated in the *Physicians' Desk Reference*. Using drugs off-label is common, however, and most physicians won't ask for a signed release form.

CHAPTER 2

Four Simple Ideas: The Topeka Tubby Diet Philosophy

First: You can't outrun your fork.

Trying to maintain weight loss through exercise is not a good long-term strategy because it's usually not sustainable. Things such as injuries, life events, and weather often interfere with a strenuous exercise program. Then weight regain will occur, because your diet is already at a moderate calorie level to sustain the exercise and prevent the hunger that comes with it. When your exercise decreases, you must go to lower calories. Because of the sponge syndrome, this becomes insidious over a period of years. Minor lapses will cause surprising weight gain.

A better strategy is to exercise less on a daily basis in a way that naturally fits into your lifestyle. A daily twenty-minute walk, for example, is sustainable for most people. Then if weight regain starts to creep in, you can engage in additional exercise on an intermittent basis to lose those three to five extra pounds. Meal replacements can also be used to make sure that overeating isn't an issue.

The reduced obese have a 42 percent reduction in their exercise metabolism, which means that a one-mile walk burns only 58 calories—not 100 calories. This adds a tremendous burden of time to what is already a difficult and challenging program just to maintain the reduced weight.

Second: The best bang for your buck for health is a twenty-minute walk.

There's no question that exercise is the fountain of youth as long as it's not overdone, but it's a poor strategy for weight loss. Significant weight loss is usually accompanied by muscle loss, although some strategies suggest that a high-protein diet combined with resistance training can prevent the muscle loss (Gretchen Reynolds, 2016, *New York Times*[14]).

There once was a belief that muscle turns into fat in muscle men, but I think those men engage in high-level exercise with high calorie intake. At some point the intense exercise stops but the intense food intake doesn't, so muscle men become overweight. Muscles burn only a small percentage of the total metabolism. Only high levels of intense performance, such as running a marathon, make a big difference. High-intensity exercise for one hour can burn 600 calories. The problem is that exercise metabolism is reduced by 38 percent after you lose 10 percent of your weight.

Resistance training is a good idea, because the muscles protect your joints from injury. Exercise for health, not for weight loss, and don't overdo it. If you're running five miles an hour and theoretically burning around 500 calories, you'll keep eating those 500 calories when you get injured and have to stop running.

Third: Weight loss usually occurs during the first six to nine months; then you plateau and regain.

This is the problem, so why don't diet books emphasize it? Instead, they talk about breaking through the plateau. Even if someone makes a monumental effort and breaks through the plateau, weight regain will occur because of low leptin levels. Fat cells shrink, but they *never disappear*. (Reference the sponge syndrome.[28]) I have broken through three plateaus—at 240 pounds, 220 pounds, and 210 pounds. I did it while following the same diet and exercise. Thanks to multiple diet medications, I felt full even though I was eating less.

To attain the initial weight loss, *virtually any low-calorie diet is acceptable*. At the plateau in six to nine months, however, I suggest switching to an ad libitum (eat until you are full) diet that you'll stay on for the rest of your life. That prevents hunger without feeling quite so restrictive.

I switched to Atkins and stopped regaining weight, despite decreasing my exercise from two and a half hours to twenty minutes per day, and I happily ate ad libitum on cruises.[7] However, I did not lose additional weight. I never could document myself to be in nutritional ketosis by urine check, probably because I did eat large amounts of food. Later I started checking my blood ketones with a finger stick and found that I was in nutritional ketosis and yet not losing weight.

Low leptin trumps ketones, exercise, and an LCHF (high-protein) diet, because it causes

- hunger,
- decreased thermogenesis (metabolism),
- increased sympathetic nervous system tone,
- delayed satiation,
- decreased perception of amount eaten,
- increased response to food,
- decreased restraint regarding food,
- decreased T3 and T4 (thyroxine), and
- increased muscle efficiency.

I believe the excess number of fat cells cause more MiRNAs to be secreted by these shrunken adipocytes with a low leptin level.[29] Hence the next step, which is unavoidable.

Fourth: Diet medications (multiple if needed)

The best way to treat low leptin levels is to take multiple diet medications. These medications fool multiple brain pathways that can cause you to gain weight despite exercise and low calorie levels. When the leptin level is low, the brain believes that the body is starving even though the patient is not yet down to his optimum weight. This is why there are two diet pills that each combine two diet medications: Qsymia (phentermine/topiramate) and Contrave (naltrexone/bupropion). The brain usually outsmarts phentermine after nine months of use.

Belviq (Locaserin) is similar to the old Fenfluramine, which caused heart valve problems that resulted in the phentermine/Fenfluramine or Fen-Phen combination being taken off the market. Unfortunately one trial showed that 50 percent of dieters don't respond to Belviq. If there is no weight loss after two months, I suggest adding phentermine at the lowest dose. This is off-label, but it's similar to the old Fen-Phen diet pill that was very effective.

Saxenda costs around $1,000 a month and most insurance doesn't cover it. So rather than putting a patient on a high dose of Saxenda, I put them on Victoza, which is covered, if they have diabetes type 2. Metformin is also covered by insurance and may help weight loss. Replacing insulin with Invokana worked well for me.

CHAPTER 3

Four New Diet Medications

Presently there are four new drugs for long-term treatment of chronic obesity. Since there is an epidemic of obesity, why isn't it being treated with medications? As a diplomat of the American Board of Obesity Medicine and a fellow and diplomat in the National Lipid Association, I think physicians should consider putting their chronically obese patients on one of the following diet medicines on a long-term basis: lorcaserin (Belviq), phentermine/topiramate (Qsymia), liraglutide (Saxenda), or naltrexone/bupropion (Contrave).

My personal experience is with Victoza, Invokana, Qsymia, and Belviq. These medications are available only with a physician's prescription. Belviq and Qsymia are controlled substances and require a physician's DEA number. I don't advise the old orlistat, because the fat-saturated diarrhea can cause terrible stains on clothes and bedsheets.

Let me give some ideas about how to choose a drug, *which must be done in concert with your physician.* Diet meds are usually indicated if BMI >26 + comorbidity or >30.

First step. If fasting glucose exceeds 99, go on metformin. This blood sugar level means that the patient has pre-diabetes. Insulin resistance (IR) is probably underdiagnosed if the insulin level is not done at the same time. If this fails to demonstrate IR, then do a two-hour postprandial glucose and insulin level to make certain you don't have insulin resistance.

Second step. If you're diabetic already and on the maximum dose of metformin, add Victoza since this low dose of liraglutide (1.8 mg) will be paid for by insurance.

Third step. If on insulin, try switching to Invokana. Carefully monitor glucose during the transition and consider switching to any low-carbohydrate, high-fat diet.[18]

Now for the diet medications themselves.

First choice? Locaserin (Belviq). This scheduled drug needs your physician's DEA number. This may be the safest drug, although patients with depression should be cautious. Young women experience fewer side effects than with Qsymia. There is a concern about serotonin syndrome, but to my knowledge this drug does not increase serotonin levels.

The downside is that only 50 percent of patients have a good response to Locaserin. However, the solution, after two or three months, is to add phentermine (one half tab, 37.5 mg per day) if you have no cardiac or anxiety contraindications. Phentermine, now available as a generic, is off-label for long term despite the combination in Qsymia having the indication for long term.

Second choice? Phentermine/topiramate (Qsymia). This scheduled drug requires your physician's DEA number. The main concern is REMS caution for pregnancy testing. It's safe for patients with depression, but in high doses it can cause cognition problems and it can taste bad, especially with diet soda. Also: potentiates alcohol, metabolic acidosis, decrease potassium, and increase creatinine. Consider getting blood chemistry levels done after the first month of treatment.

Third choice? Naltrexone/bupropion (Contrave). This is a nonscheduled drug, so a physician's DEA number isn't required. The bad news is label legacy. These two drugs have been around for so long that many side effects have shown up in the *Physicians' Desk Reference* over the years. The black box warning concerns patients with depression and neuro-psych disorders. This medication shouldn't be taken by people on narcotic pain medicine or patients with bulimia or anorexia nervosa. Caution should be exercised with patients prone to seizures, and this might not be a good choice for young folks who might binge on alcohol. Don't take this medication with Levadopa or amantadine. There are still some concerns about increased hypertension or high blood pressure, and constipation tends to occur with weight loss but seems worse with Contrave.

Fourth choice? Liraglutide (Saxenda). This is a nonscheduled drug, so a physician's DEA number isn't required. Taken by injection, this drug is expensive. Diabetics can get a lower dose paid for as Victoza. The black box warning concerns thyroid C cell tumors. Side effects include vomiting, pancreatitis, and abdominal pain. Forty percent of people complain about this drug, but they usually tough it out and stay on it.

How does bariatric surgery work? Surprise! Not by restricting the amount of food the body can take in. Surgery works much like diet medications. Using hormones, it fools the brain into thinking that it's not hungry on a reduced diet. Frank Greenway wrote, in a recent review of obesity medicine, "Following gastric bypass surgery, levels of ghrelin are extremely low, while GLP-1 and PYY are elevated, which should attenuate appetite."[19]

Choosing which weight loss surgery is best for a patient is not based on random controlled double-blind trials. Lap band was the most popular, but it doesn't work as well in the long term because it's not a bypass surgery. It only restricts the amount of food in the stomach. Surgeons are allowed the freedom to determine the best course for obese patients without random controlled trials, whereas medical physicians face possible state sanctions while searching for the best diet medication combination for their patients.

ABOM (American Board of Obesity Medicine) specialists need to be allowed to use the best off-label treatment with multiple drugs to block the multiple pathways of starvation prevention that cause weight regain. Use of multiple off-label drugs is already being done to treat type 2 diabetes mellitus, high blood pressure, and infectious disease. When leptin is low, it does not inhibit ghrelin, which is activated and increases hunger.

CHAPTER 4

No False Hope Here

Gina Kolata introduced me to the idea of false hope in her 2007 book *Rethinking Thin.*[20] I quoted from several of her chapters in my 2011 book, *The Tubby Traveler from Topeka.*[7] The idea that diet and exercise alone will maintain weight loss is still being advised in the guidelines. This is a false hope that is achieved by only a few members of the National Weight Control Registry, who are maintaining a 1,200 to 1,500 calorie diet with one hour of exercise per day.[31] This is a sub-starvation diet just to maintain weight loss. The reason it's not a starvation diet is that the low leptin levels prevent starvation with the sponge syndrome.[34]

The reduced obese must find a restrictive diet they can stay on for the rest of their lives. High-density carbs in large quantities will sabotage any diet, even along with diet medications and strenuous exercise or following bariatric surgery. We are indefensible against unlimited M&M's or excess alcohol.

The key to a sustainable diet is to not be hungry. More exercise makes you more hungry. This is why more exercise is not the answer to maintaining weight loss, unless you maintain the same 1,200 to 1,500 calories a day as the people in the NWCR do. When the volunteers in the Great Starvation diet did this for twenty-four weeks, they suffered terribly.[4] Dr. Aronne believes his intense exercise will not have this effect, as it is only ten minutes twice a week. We will see how it works out for his patients.[2] However, exercising to muscle failure is too intense for most patients and will cause injury, in my opinion.

Atkins (ad libitum) and very-low-calorie diets (VLCD) of 800 to 1,000 calories say that the subsequent nutritional ketosis these diets cause results in less appetite. As with many attempts (high protein and nutritional ketosis) to decrease hunger, eventually a diet medication should be added after six to nine months, when the body will compensate with more hunger as the brain thinks it is starving because of the low leptin level. David Ludwig, in *Always Hungry,* believes that low-glycemic carbohydrates will not stimulate insulin release that results in less hunger.[1]

Bariatric surgery, excluding lap bands, does not really work on restricting food amount. It works on hormonal changes in the gut that tell your brain that you're full. Sadly, these are all short-term solutions when looking at ten-year data. Thirty percent of people gain their weight back ten years after bariatric surgery.[35]

CHAPTER 5

The Science of Obesity

Insulin is probably one of the main reasons people gain their weight back from the plateau of weight loss. Let me go through the physiology.

Insulin peripherally is *anabolic*. It promotes constructive metabolism. Insulin will store fat in adipose and glycogen in muscle and liver. Insulin centrally is *catabolic*. Like leptin, insulin breaks down molecules to release energy.

Low leptin increases food intake and suppresses energy expenditure. "Leptin is an important signal for starvation" (Youdim, p. 6). *High* leptin reduces food intake by inhibiting NPY/AgRP neurons and stimulating the alpha-MSH neurons, *except in the obese* who become *leptin resistant*. Only lean individuals appear to be regulating body weight.

Centrally, leptin and insulin share same feeding inhibitory and thermogenic pathways. "However, in obese, insulin triggers steroidogenic factor 1 (SF-1) expressing neurons of the VMH, resulting in inhibition of POMC neurons, which promotes food intake and perpetuates obesity."[21]

Let me repeat: In lean people who have never been obese, leptin and insulin prevent them from becoming obese. *Centrally* high levels of leptin and insulin reduce food intake and suppress energy expenditure through the same pathway. Centrally both insulin and leptin are catabolic. When a lean person eats a large meal, a high level of insulin from the pancreas peripherally stores fat and adipose and centrally increases thermogenesis to burn excess calories to maintain weight.

A "genetically obese prone" person with early insulin resistance and early leptin resistance does all of this less effectively. They store more fat, burn less energy, and allow more food intake, on their way down the slippery slope of always more appetite and more fat with more leptin and insulin resistance.

With tremendous willpower, an obese person who follows the 3,500 calorie rule—cut 3,500 calories to lose one pound of weight per week—will be able to lose weight for six to nine months. Then they'll reach the plateau, the thermodynamic laws of physics will fail, and the biological laws of survival will take over and their body will tell them that they're starving.

The plethora of retained fat cells in the reduced obese give the brain this early warning even before a person reaches their desired normal BMI, which is typically their weight when they graduated from high school or got married. Fat cells don't disappear—they shrink. The subsequent low leptin level in the face of so many fat cells signals the body that starvation is occurring by sending out MiRNAs from an increased number of fat cells.[29] This is the *sponge syndrome.*

According to Michael Hopkin, "Fat cell numbers stay constant through adult life. Even serious weight loss doesn't reduce your overall number of fat-holding cells."[28] The reduced obese have so many fat cells, but so little leptin. Their insulin is probably high, but they are resistant to its glucose-lowering effect. MiRNAs are sent from the fat cells throughout the body via the blood stream (episomes).

The body's first priority is to conserve energy by not heating the body, so that the lower-calorie diet can be used to restore fat cells to their previous size. Thermogenesis is reduced in the plateau, as the determined dieter drops to 800 calories or increases to three hours of walking every day. At this point, the physics of the 3,500 calorie rule fail.

This is when the dieter learns that most of the calories that they're burning are being used by their resting metabolism. Up to 70 percent of calories may be burned by the brain, liver, kidneys, heart, lungs, and endocrine organs, and the brain alone burns 25 percent of total calories. Muscles themselves become food at this point, rather than the tool by which a weight lifter loses weight. *Thermogenesis is reduced by leptin, insulin, and probably MiRNA*, but the dieter can do nothing about this. Could the new diet pills and a gastric bypass help?

Introducing ghrelin, the only hormone that stimulates the appetite.

Leptin inhibits ghrelin, but not in obese people; likewise, insulin inhibits ghrelin centrally, but not in obese people. The reduced obese, with their billions of excess shrunken fat cells and subsequent low leptin levels, have high ghrelin levels. These people can think about nothing except their next meal. This sub-starvation state, a miserable psychological condition, is where most diet guidelines and books tell us we must stay to maintain our weight loss. They are wrong. This condition is not sustainable.[14]

High insulin levels will take any food we eat and use it for fat storage. It might take years, but at any moment of mild excess food intake above 1,000 calories, those extra calories will be used to store fat—*not* to build muscle or generate body heat. Surviving the famine is the body's main objective. The sponge of excess fat cells, with the help of insulin, will convert food to fat at low levels of calorie intake to slowly raise the leptin level back to a safe level for survival. MiRNAs probably also play a key role, though that is yet to be conclusively determined.

Ochner writes in 2015, "Additional biological adaptations occur with the development of obesity and these function to preserve, or even increase, an individual's highest sustained lifetime bodyweight. For example, preadipocyte proliferation occurs, increasing fat storage capacity."[22]

This is why you can't maintain weight loss and your plateau usually isn't even close to your optimum BMI. Your body uses your leptin level to determine your risk of starvation. Your reduced obese body has the same number of fat cells as your former maximum obese self, and all those excess shrunken fat cells secrete an excess of MiRNA. Your body uses the adipocytes that it has, and they never go away. If you surgically remove them, they grow back somewhere else. Brain cells can die, but fat cells replace themselves because they are more important for survival.

Obese people are leptin resistant and often insulin resistant, so leptin and insulin act differently in the obese state. They also act differently in the reduced obese state, which is why people cannot maintain weight loss despite low calorie diets and exercise. The answer is that there is a convergence of evidence from multiple lines of inquiry.

Part of the anorexic (feeding inhibitory) pathway:

- Leptin
- Insulin
- Ileal brake, a form of gut traffic management, controls the rate at which food moves through the gut.
- Locaserin (Belviq) activates POMC neurons in the brain.
- Alpha MSH release

Part of feed stimulatory pathway:

- Ghrelin opposes leptin effect in hypothalamus; leptin inhibits ghrelin action.
- Ghrelin activates NPY/AgRP neuron.
- Ghrelin stimulates the release of NPY and AgRP.

Medications were designed to affect these pathways. Because the brain compensates for one medication, multiple medications are needed to affect many of the different pathways.

CHAPTER 6

Treatment of Chronic Obesity

My approach is for a patient to lose weight on any diet that has worked for them before. I suggest they continue the same exercise they were doing before the diet. If they injure themselves in the middle of a diet, the decrease in exercise will sabotage the program.

The diet book industry does very well because any reduction in calories will work in the six-to-nine-month period of weight loss before the plateau kicks in. Ochner writes, "Many clinicians are not adequately aware of the reasons that individuals with obesity struggle to achieve and maintain weight loss, and this poor awareness precludes the provision of effective intervention."[22]

When does the disease of chronic obesity start? Dr. Aronne suggests that if you have been yo-yo dieting for years, you have chronic obesity.[2] In this epidemic of obesity, I suspect that if your BMI is at 30 or above, and then you lose 10 percent of your weight, you become one of the reduced obese with billions of shrunken fat cells. Then the sponge syndrome kicks in, your low leptin level constantly tells your brain that you're starving, and your excess fat cells release MiRNA to cause weight regain even at a low calorie level. It's the huge number of adipocytes (fat cells) that cause weight regain, and slowly increasing low glycemic foods in the reduced obese will *not* "reprogram" the fat cells, as Dr. Ludwig suggests in his book, *Always Hungry*.[1]

The solution.

- Exercise: Walk twenty minutes a day for health, not for weight loss.
- Diet: Stay on an ad libitum diet that does not allow you to be hungry.
- Diet medication: Once you hit the plateau and become one of the reduced obese, take medications that will help you maintain your weight loss and perhaps help you lose more weight.

To keep a patient on a diet medicine without clinical benefit (or 5 percent weight loss) is probably off-label. An obesity physician should not be restricted by a rule that fails to recognize that individual patients need multiple diet medications to cover multiple pathways of weight regain. If the obese patient experiences reduced joint pain or better blood pressure or glucose levels, then I believe the rules permit keeping that patient on that diet medication for the rest of their lives, even if they don't hit the 5 percent weight loss mark.

First Diet Suggestion: Atkins

Atkins (LCHF) is an ad libitum diet, which means that you eat until you're full. Because of habit and cravings, it's difficult for the obese to realize when they are full and then stop eating even when on diet medications. Liraglutide may cause a person to vomit because of delayed stomach emptying. Many people believe that carbohydrates increase insulin, which increases hunger in two to three hours.

Advantages to Atkins:

- No calorie counting
- Fat (butter, mayonnaise, etc.) makes food taste good.
- Protein satisfies appetite.
- Easy to follow; just don't eat carbohydrates.

Second Diet Suggestion: KISS (Keep It Simple, Stupid)

The first goal with the KISS diet is to keep it simple and use prepared meals to calculate calories accurately. Atkins frozen meals are okay, or you can use protein shakes or bars. People on very low calorie diets of 800 calories can usually get expensive prepared meals through their diet physicians.

The second goal is to put the patient in nutritional ketosis with high protein to prevent hunger, although this might not end cravings. If you don't get a positive urine strip for ketone after two to three weeks, try blood strips for ketones and finger sticks. If still not in ketosis, try to fast for one or two days.

If you can keep carbs down to six days a week and not binge on them, the Atkins diet might still work for you. You may have to wait up to twelve months before you allow yourself a carb night. If I bring ice cream or a whole pizza into the house, I can't limit my portions. If I don't eat at least 30 grams of protein at breakfast, lunch, and dinner, I get hungry between meals. Then I eat a protein snack that has at least 10 grams of protein. The Atkins French vanilla shake is 160 calories, 2g CHO (carbs), and 15 grams protein. I also eat almonds or pistachios.

Even with the high-protein diet, the more I exercise, the hungrier I get. Diet medication allows me to eat less on the same Atkins diet and exercise but still lose weight. Diet medication has also allowed me to not regain on the same diet and exercise without increased hunger.

If you're unable to lose weight or you need a short-term diet because you're regaining, try the KISS diet. It's not ad libitum, but if you're motivated, you can be successful in the short term, and diet medications can help to prevent your hunger. The following KISS diet has 65 percent fat.

		Calories	Protein	Carbs
Breakfast	3 eggs	465	27g	0g
Snack	Atkins vanilla shake	160	15g	2g

		Calories	Protein	Carbs
Lunch	Atkins frozen meal (beef in merlot)	310	20g	10g
Snack	Atkins vanilla shake	160	15g	2g
Dinner	Beef fillet 6 oz.	414	44g	0g
	Blue cheese dressing (2 tbsp) with salad	150	1g	1g
Snack	Light and Lively Greek Yogurt	80	12g	9g
Total		1739	134g	24g

Also you should stay hydrated. If you get cramps or feel weak, drink chicken bouillon for salt replacement. Add magnesium too, but make sure that you don't have renal insufficiency. Take a multivitamin, and add low-calorie Metamucil if you're constipated. Walk at least twenty minutes per day, or eight minutes after each meal.

I suggest the KISS diet only for the short term, if your diet or Atkins ad libitum isn't working, to help you lose weight or maintain weight loss. You may get hungry on this diet, since it's calorie restricted and not ad libitum.

Third Diet Suggestion: Bon Vivant

The bon vivant diet allows you to eat until you're full and avoid feeling hungry. It allows one to two ounces of alcohol per day. You might find that you lose willpower with alcohol, but it decreases my cravings, especially when I have it after dinner for dessert. Avoid being sedentary, but exercise is not strenuous—a twenty-minute, one-mile walk per day is sufficient.

This is a substantial change, but it's a change that can be maintained for life with the help of diet medications, because the drugs fight off the hunger of decreased leptin and increased MiRNA. Ultimately, the treatment of the reduced obese's low level of leptin will be multiple diet medications, since there are multiple hormonal pathways to prevent you from starving.

CHAPTER 7

What Doctors Read About Low-Carbohydrate Diets

I bought a $500 subscription to UpToDate.com for the latest information on medical science. This is what I got for my money on low-carbohydrate diets:

Obesity in adults: Dietary therapy
Author: George A Bray, MD et al.

All topics are updated (on UpToDate.com) as new evidence becomes available and our peer review process is complete.
Literature review current through: Jul 2016. This topic last updated: Jun 15, 2016.

"Low- and very-low-carbohydrate diets are more effective for short-term weight loss than low-fat diets, although probably not for long-term weight loss. A meta-analysis of five trials found that the difference in weight loss at six months, favoring the low-carbohydrate over low-fat diet, was not sustained at 12 months."

A good head-to-head two-year trial is the Shai trial. Head-to-head diets of low-fat, Mediterranean, and low-carb diets were compared. LCHF diets resulted in the most weight loss after two years.

It's not clear to me why the UpToDate.com review did not give this reference credence.

CHAPTER 8

Nutritional Ketosis: Are Ketogenic Diets Better at Weight Loss?

I have presented two excellent scientific articles on obesity, the Greenway article[19] and the Ochner article,[22] in which nutritional ketosis is never discussed. In my Obesity Board training, I was taught that very low calorie diets (VLCD) of fewer than 1,000 calories usually result in nutritional ketosis, which suppresses appetite.

Surprise Secret Weapon of Diets: Meal Replacements

To my surprise, the most effective way to lose weight is meal replacements, which are also useful in maintaining weight. I eat Atkins meals because they're high in protein and low in carbs. Eating prepared meals prevents you from underestimating your daily calorie count. Using meal replacements for a short time when you have a minor weight gain might be helpful.

Simplicity is key to the treatment of chronic obesity, and fancy recipes decrease compliance. Prepared meals with an exact number of calories are the perfect tool for lifelong dieters at various times in our ever-changing, stressful lives. My problem was that my hunger wasn't at all satisfied with one prepared meal, but diet medications have eliminated that problem.

Prepared meals are satisfying in very low calorie diets when patients are in nutritional ketosis and their hunger is blunted. Unfortunately, when reduced obese reach the plateau and the sponge syndrome kicks in, nutritional ketosis and protein satiation are not enough. The low leptin level from their shrunken fat cells will make the reduced obese want to eat several meal replacements, even though these meals are high in protein and low in carbohydrates.

When a reduced obese patient has to walk 10,000 steps a day to break through the plateau, their hunger is incredible and a meal replacement will not suffice. But when the reduced obese walk just one mile a day for health, if they notice a weight regain, meal replacements are a perfect way to make certain their portion size isn't getting too large, and diet medications will also help minimize their hunger. Price is an issue, but this is still cheaper than gastric bypass surgery.

CHAPTER 9

Can You Preserve Muscle Mass with Weight Loss?

You can't outrun your fork. But maybe with certain weight lifting programs and 2.4g/kg per day of protein, the obese can use lean body weight.

"In summary, the present study provides evidence that, in young men, consuming a higher protein diet (2.4g·kg–1·d–1) during energy deficit (~40% reduction in energy intake compared with requirements) while performing intense resistance exercise training and HIT can augment LBM over a 28-d period. Furthermore, these high-intensity exercises performed during a period of energy deficit have the ability to preserve LBM despite a lower protein intake (1.2g·kg–1·d–1). In conclusion, the current study provides direct evidence that a higher protein diet during substantial energy deficit and HIT not only preserves, but increases, LBM and HIT during the energy deficit, irrespective of protein intake, and increases strength and performance in young men."[24]

"We provide novel evidence of the effect of lifting markedly different (lighter vs. heavier) loads (mass per repetition) during whole-body resistance training on the development of muscle strength and hypertrophy in previously trained persons. Using a large sample size (n = 49), and contradicting dogma, we report that the relative load lifted per repetition does not determine skeletal muscle hypertrophy or, for the most part, strength development. In line with our previous work, acute postexercise systemic hormonal changes were unrelated to strength and hypertrophic gains."[25]

My first bioelectrical weight was done at the Los Angeles obesity conference on November 6, 2015. It helped me follow muscle loss that occurs with weight loss. Now that I'm at a plateau of 200 pounds, I'm trying to increase muscle. I suspect I will gain some weight on 150 grams of protein, but I hope to keep my fat percentage down.

In 2015, I gained muscle on Atkins while in nutritional ketosis. Spending one hour per day on weight lifting and walking, and consuming extra protein, I went from 238 pounds on May 3 to 244.5 pounds on June 23. (Weight checked on home scale, no breakfast, no clothes.)

June 23, 2015
Bioelectrical Impedance Scale
Weight 244.8 with clothes

Total H2O 49.9%
Total body fat 31%
Fat-free mass 68.9%
Muscle mass 46.1 lb.

June 24, 2015
Started Qsymia 3.75/23 mg and stopped weight lifting

December 11, 2015
Bioelectrical Impedance Scale[26]
Weight 222.4 (lost 22.4 lb.)
Total H2O 53.2%
Total body fat 26.6% (dropped 4.4%)
Fat-free mass 71.8
Muscle mass 41.8 (dropped 4.3 lb.)

The second Gretchen Reynolds article from the *New York Times*[27] suggests three sets of low-weight lifting at twenty-five reps four times a week. In my 65-year-old body, I found getting to twenty-five repetitions quite difficult even at the lowest weight. Elderly men develop sarcopenia mostly with muscle loss in their legs, so I try to do some leg weight lifting.

The Aronne (Zickerman) method of two ten-minute workouts a week to achieve absolute muscle failure seems guaranteed to cause injury, despite their advice to go super slow. It's the final ten seconds of going for the burn that worries me, because that's the injury zone. This workout method is better designed for young people.

In the summer of 2015, I increased my exercise by about 300 percent. I doubled my walks to forty minutes a day, did circuit weight lifting two or three days per week, and did water aerobics two or three days per week. I ate more and gained two pounds, one-half pound of which was muscle.

	Weight	Fat %	Muscle	H20	BMI
6-15-16	219.8	26.8%	41.3 lb.	54.1%	30.4
7-20-16	221.6	27.2%	41.7 lb.	53.7%	30.7

Let's see what happens with more protein and Gretchen's four sets of twenty-five reps of light weights four times a week:

How much protein for each person? A total of 2.4 grams of protein for each kg of lean body weight. It's difficult to figure lean body weight without a bioelectrical impedance scale.

    5-1-17:   Weight = 204 lb. (92.5 kg)
                 Fat = 24.9% (22.8 kg)

Subtract 22.8 (total fat) from 92.5 (total body weight) = 69.7 (lean body weight)
Thus for me: 2.4 x 69.7 = 167.08 grams of protein per day.

My diet yesterday:

		Protein	Calories	Carbs	Fiber
Breakfast	3 eggs fried in butter	18g	300	0	0
	3 slices bacon	9g	165	0	0
	Butter 1 tbsp		100		
Lunch	Atkins Beef	16g	310	9g	3g
	Almonds 28 nuts	6g	170	6g	3g
	Premium Protein	30g	160	2g	
Dinner	Tenderloin filet 7 oz	56g	490	0	0
	Cauliflower 1 oz	0.5	14	1.0	
	Butter 1 tbsp		100		
	Pistachios I/2 cup	6g	160	8g	3g
	Light and Lively yogurt	12g	80	9g	0
	Red wine 12 oz	0	240	6g	
Totals		153g	2599	41g	9g

"Total dietary fiber intake should be 25 to 30 grams a day from food, not supplements. Currently, dietary fiber intakes among adults in the United States average about 15 grams a day" (UCSF Medical Center).

I doubt this is important unless you're constipated.

CHAPTER 10

Evidence for Weight Loss Maintenance with Exercise

How strong is the evidence that exercise is effective for weight loss and weight loss maintenance? Paul Maclean, from Innovative Research, answers this question with data I took from his slide at the Fall Obesity Summit plenary sessions in 2015:

- Two trials found benefit to exercise in weight loss maintenance: Jeffery 2003 and Pavlou 1986.
- Eight trials found no benefit to exercise in weight loss maintenance: Wing 1998, Tate 2007, Skender 1996, Fogelholm 2000, Perri 1986, Leemarkers 1999, Borg 2002, and Jakicic 2008.

The NLA guideline chart does not specifically address exercise advice for maintaining weight loss.

CHAPTER 11

Sponge Syndrome in the Reduced Obese

Can you eat 7 calories per pound and walk five miles every day of your life to maintain your weight? This is how the people in the National Weight Registry Program maintained their weight loss over five years. The guidelines are based on the success of the reduced obese who have lost thirty pounds and maintained that weight loss over five years. If those ten thousand people could do it, then the rest of us should be able to do it. However, for people with chronic obesity, the sponge syndrome makes it difficult.

Who has chronic obesity?

If you lost more than 10 percent of your body weight, but then gained it back over the next five to ten years despite your best efforts, you have chronic obesity. Also sometimes called yo-yo dieting, chronic obesity is caused by the sponge syndrome. Once a person reaches a BMI of 30, there are simply too many fat cells that never go away.

What is the sponge syndrome?

I first wrote about the sponge syndrome in my 2012 book, *The Tubby Traveler from Topeka*.[7] No matter how much weight you lose, fat cells don't disappear—they just shrink.

"Fat cell numbers stay constant through adult life," says Michael Hopkin. "Even serious weight loss doesn't reduce your overall number of fat-holding cells. The researchers also measured 20 people who were obese and had 'stomach stapling' surgery to reduce food intake. When Spalding and her team measured these volunteers again two years after the procedure, they found no reduction in fat-cell number: the subjects still had over 80 billion individual fat cells in their bodies, Spalding and her colleagues calculate. Nevertheless, fat cells are constantly dying and being replaced, even in adults, Spalding and her team found."[28]

Low in leptin, these adipocytes tell your brain that you're starving. This happens before you reach your optimum BMI or body weight, because your brain anticipates starvation before all your fat is gone. Losing a large amount of fat isn't good for survival, so leptin starts sending messages to your brain before you hit your target weight. MiRNA, packaged as episomes via the bloodstream, is also sent out from the adipocytes to the cells of the body to help regain weight.

My sponge syndrome theory, based on low leptin levels in lifelong cells, was supported in "Long-Term Persistence of Hormonal Adaptations to Weight Loss," by Priya Sumithran, which I quote in *The Tubby Traveler from Topeka*:[7]

> Worldwide, there are more than 1.5 billion overweight adults, including 400 million who are obese. Although dietary restriction often results in initial weight loss, the majority of obese dieters fail to maintain their reduced weight. Understanding the barriers to maintenance of weight loss is crucial for the prevention of relapse. Body weight is centrally regulated, with peripheral hormonal signals released from the gastrointestinal tract, pancreas, and adipose tissue integrated, primarily in the hypothalamus, to regulate food intake and energy expenditure. The number of identified peripheral modulators of appetite is expanding rapidly and includes leptin, ghrelin, cholecystokinin, peptide YY, insulin, pancreatic polypeptide, and glucagon-like peptide 1 (GLP-1). Caloric restriction results in acute compensatory changes, including profound reductions in energy expenditure, levels of leptin, cholecystokinin, and increases in ghrelin and appetite, all of which promote weight regain.[36]

When leptin is low, it doesn't inhibit ghrelin, which is activated and then increases hunger. Leptin and insulin share the same central feeding inhibitory and thermogenic pathways. Peripherally insulin is anabolic, storing fat in adipose and glycogen in muscle and liver. Centrally insulin, like leptin, is catabolic, which means that it breaks down molecules to release energy. Insulin resistance is seen in prediabetes (fasting glucose of 100 or greater), metabolic syndrome (waist greater than 40 inches causing high visceral fat), and diabetes mellitus type 2.

Insulin resistance impairs the capacity of the insulin receptor to signal the fat cell to halt triglyceride breakdown by lipase and increases glucose uptake by glucose transport proteins. This increases the release of fatty acids into central circulation and decreases the uptake of glucose by fat cells.

Once again Gina Kolata puts a spotlight on the false hope of diet and exercise in her *New York Times* article on May 2, 2016, "After *The Biggest Loser*, Their Bodies Fought to Regain Weight":

> Researchers knew that just about anyone who deliberately loses weight—even if they start at a normal weight or even underweight—will have a slower metabolism when the diet ends. So they were not surprised to see that *The Biggest Loser* contestants had slow metabolisms when the show ended. What shocked the researchers was what happened next: As the years went by and the numbers on the scale climbed, the contestants' metabolisms did not recover. They became even slower, and the pounds kept piling on. It was as if their bodies were intensifying their effort to pull the contestants back to their original weight. Mr. Cahill was one of the worst off. As he regained more than 100 pounds, his metabolism slowed so much that, just to maintain his current weight of 295 pounds, he now has to eat 800 calories a day less than a typical man his size. Anything more turns to fat.[14]

This research validated my sponge syndrome theory that the reduced obese suffer from fifty types of obesity simplified to three types: (1) never obese, (2) reduced obese with prediabetes or metabolic syndrome or diabetes, and (3) reduced obese without high sugar or metabolic syndrome.

There are many genes that predispose to obesity but are not guaranteed to cause it. Some rare diseases are clearly caused by genetics, such as Bardet-Biedl syndrome and Prader-Willi syndrome, but other more common diseases also can cause obesity:

- Hypothyroidism can be treated with thyroid medication.
- Polycystic ovary syndrome (PCOS) has been effectively treated with metformin.
- Cushing's syndrome produces excess steroids in the body.

Some medications—psychiatric, anti-seizure, diabetic, contraceptive, protease inhibitors, antihistamines, antihypertensives, and so on—cause weight gain. Fortunately these classes of drugs usually include some specific medications that don't cause obesity.

"Obesity, however, is not unique in causing WAT (white adipose tissue) remodeling. Changes in adiposity also occur with aging, calorie restriction, cancers, and diseases such as HIV infection."[37]

Lipodystrophy

As an infectious disease specialist, I have seen HIV patients with lipodystrophy. At a conference many years ago, someone suggested that if we find the cause of lipodystrophy, we might use it to treat obesity. Lipodystrophy, however, is not a pretty way to lose weight. "Lipodystrophy is a medical condition characterized by abnormal or degenerative conditions of the body's adipose tissue … This condition is also characterized by a lack of circulating leptin which may lead to osteosclerosis." (from Wiki)

Insulin resistance impairs the capacity of the insulin receptor to signal the fat cell to halt triglyceride breakdown by lipase and increases glucose uptake by glucose transport proteins. This increases the release of fatty acids into central circulation and decreases the uptake of glucose by fat cells. In lean people, insulin reduces food uptake by inhibiting NPY/AgRP neurons (unidirectional). But in the obese, insulin triggers the steroidogenic factor (SF-1), which promotes food intake and perpetuates obesity.
"CNS insulin signaling in the control of energy homeostasis."[21]

"The action of insulin on the Reward Pathway Dopaminergic is thought to contribute to development of obesity, since signaling of these higher neuronal circuits can override hypothalamic signaling. High sugar or high fat diet leads to neuronal insulin resistance and dysregulation of dopamine homeostasis and dopamine homeostasis leading to hypodopaminergic reward deficit syndrome."[38]

CHAPTER 12

Sponge Syndrome Validation

I believe my sponge syndrome theory explains the main cause of chronic obesity, as verified by multiple scientific discoveries. We don't know what has caused the growing obesity epidemic. Gaining and losing weight is relatively easy, but maintaining weight loss is the challenge.

The guidelines advise to maintain weight loss with more exercise and limit caloric intake to 1,000 to 1,500, depending on your height. However, this strategy has worked for only about 5 percent of the chronically obese over the long term.[31] The leptin hormonal theory of weight regain in the reduced obese has clearly been elucidated.[17] The leptin theory has also been validated by many medications that fool leptin by telling your brain that it's not starving via several different hormonal pathways downstream from leptin.

It's a fact that weight loss and bariatric surgery do not reduce the number of fat cells. Instead, they cause shrinkage of the adipocytes with subsequent low levels of leptin, which act directly on the brain.[28] It's also a fact that small fat cells are more efficient at gaining weight in reduced obese.[22] There are leptin receptors throughout the body, and adipocytes also send out MiRNAs to tell the body via episomes to regain weight.[29]

Most diet books ignore all this science. As Dr. Aronne reminds us, it takes new science up to fourteen years to accept new data. Although the term *nutrition science* might be considered an oxymoron, we've seen three good nutrition science trials in the past few years: the PREDIMED trial, the Look AHEAD trial, and the DASH diet trial to treat hypertension. Unfortunately we don't know if the secret sauce in the PREDIMED is wine, and nutritionists discount the Look AHEAD negative outcomes.

"Consilience of inductions. Call it a "convergence of evidence"[23] not found for low fat diet despite multiple trials and not found for exercise to maintain weight loss. (See chapter 10.)

I pushed the sponge syndrome theory as a commonsense answer to why people regain their weight loss. What the nutritionists and the guidelines push to maintain weight loss has not worked. To continue giving weight loss advice that doesn't work for 80 to 95 percent of the reduced obese might be called insanity.

Resistance to low-carbohydrate, high-fat (LCHF) diets has been fierce, but there is finally a paradigm shift. Studies have shown that some people do better on low-fat diets, but overall the data for LCHF is excellent. Is it genetics or cultural? Shifting from a high- to a low-carb diet is difficult, but it is possible if you stick with Atkins (LCHF) long enough to get over your love of carbohydrates, which takes at least a month. I suspect the difficulty is more cultural than genetic, but time will tell.

I want people to lose weight with whatever diet has worked for them in the past. Once they hit their plateau, low-fat diets fail in the long run because they aren't ad libitum. People can stay on a diet for life only if the diet satiates their hunger via high protein and nutritional ketosis. Also, fat gives food much of its flavor. You need to follow a reduced-calorie diet that you can stay on for the rest of your life just to maintain your weight loss, although you won't lose additional weight.

No matter what diet you go on, eventually it will fail because a diet can't reduce the number of fat cells in your body. Only diet medications can overcome the low leptin levels that tell your brain that your body is starving.[35] This science isn't often mentioned in articles on weight loss maintenance. I've tried to present some of it without getting too much into the weeds and keeping it as simple as possible. I took the American Board of Obesity Medicine boards, but unfortunately other disciplines don't know or won't accept this data.

Thus "convergence of evidence" went awry during the decades of low-fat dieting. Possibly the influence of food production lobbyists had something to do with it. For example, Dr. Ludwig writes that guidelines allowing fruit juices might have to do with lobby interests on the guideline board in his tweets: "The 2015 to 2020 Dietary Guidelines for Americans (DGAs) recognize the role of 100% fruit juice in health and in helping people meet daily fruit recommendations and state that 100% fruit juice is a nutrient-dense beverage that should be a primary choice, along with water and low-fat/fat-free milk."[39] For my sponge syndrome theory "to overturn the consensus, I would need to find flaws with all the lines of supportive evidence and show a consistent convergence of evidence toward a different theory that explains the data."[23]

The Hall analysis of *The Biggest Loser* puts a big question mark next to advice regarding exercise and low calorie intake, since that did not work for thirteen of fifteen people in the trial.[14] The Look AHEAD data showed that after ten years of the best exercise and diet program with close personal support, behavioral changes failed in primary outcomes compared with control. This was a random controlled trial with a large number of participants and a good control over ten years. It doesn't get much better than this in nutrition science. Yet this data did not change the guidelines, most of which still advise ninety minutes or more of exercise to maintain weight. (See chapter 13.)

The key to maintaining weight loss is diet medications and a low-calorie, ad libitum diet that you can stay on the rest of your life. No guidelines should be written without a close examination of the many ways the brain uses hormones to make you gain weight again. The sponge syndrome is the perfect storm for weight regain in the reduced obese.[34] The number of fat cells has the last word. I asked Dr. Leibel if adipocytes live only ten years, but he said there is evidence that the fat cells that die are rapidly replaced. Thus the billions of excess fat cells are present for life in the reduced obese and act like a sponge for free fatty acids.

I had the privilege of hearing Dr. Michael Rosenbaum talk about why weight loss maintenance is so difficult. I asked him if what I call the sponge syndrome might also make it difficult to maintain weight loss. Small fat cells are efficient at regaining fat, and the reduced obese have a large number of fat cells despite their weight loss. He asked why skinny people with skinny fat cells don't regain weight as well. I don't think he understood that I was referring to the reduced obese, who have a much higher leptin threshold than a lean person who was never fat and whose small fat cells are not increased in number.

Similar to the Frank Greenway review,[19] I was gratified to find that the Ochner review supported much of my theory that the sponge syndrome is a contributing factor in the chronic disease of obesity: "Irrespective of starting weight, caloric restriction triggers several biological adaptations designed to prevent starvation. These adaptations might be potent enough to undermine the long-term effectiveness of lifestyle modification in most individuals with obesity, particularly in an environment that promotes energy overconsumption."[22]

Ochner says that preadipocyte proliferation increases fat storage capacity. This goes along with what I hypothesized in my sponge syndrome theory. As Ochner says, "These biological adaptations often persist indefinitely, even when a person re-attains a healthy BMI via behaviourally induced weight loss."[3] Ochner goes on to say that "few individuals ever truly recover from obesity; individuals who formerly had obesity but are able to re-attain a healthy body weight via diet and exercise still have 'obesity in remission.'"

CHAPTER 13

Look AHEAD: The Biggest Failure of Diet and Exercise

Look AHEAD was a negative-outcome trial of the best that diet and exercise could do for a control group over ten years.[10] Here's the data that every weight loss diet book should present: a 2.5 percent weight loss compared with control. After ten years of work and suffering, a 2.5 percent improvement over the control is the best that could be achieved?

Look AHEAD had the usual waterfall weight loss results that show up in any diet trial. Of the treated group, 39.3 percent did maintain >10 percent weight loss, which is great. However, 17.2 percent of the control group had >10 percent weight loss after eight years. Remember, half of the people in the National Weight Control Registry maintain their weight loss on their own. A great deal of money was spent over ten years to counsel the treatment group with little effect and a negative trial outcome.

According to the *New England Journal of Medicine*,[41] "Weight loss was greater in the intervention group than the control group throughout (8.6% vs. 0.7% at 1 year; 6.0% vs. 3.5% at study end)." That's a 2.5 percent difference.

Surgery creates false hope, because it's actually all about adaptive thermogenesis. Shrunken fat cells don't disappear, and the low leptin level eventually causes the body to regain weight. Thirty percent of bariatric surgery patients regain all their weight after ten years. Even gastric bypass surgeries have waterfall results, with many patients gaining weight comparing two-year results with six-year results.[35]

In the sponge syndrome, billions of shrunken fat cells cause weight regain after six to nine months of weight loss because of leptin deficiency.

CHAPTER 14

Bioelectrical Impedance Scale

I had my body fat determined by calipers on skin fat on March 27, 1997. At 45 years of age, I weighed 242 pounds and had a 45-inch waist. My computed body fat was 27 percent, I had 65 pounds of fat, and my lean body weight was calculated at 177. I think this undercalculated my body fat percentage. Perhaps I had much more muscle mass, but a caliper test did not measure that.

At age 47, I tried to join the Reserves. They did not use calipers.

- Weight 240 pounds
- Waist 48 inches
- Neck circumference 17.5 inches
- Abdominal-neck factor 113.49
- Height factor 80.25
- Subtract height factor from abdominal-neck factor = 33.24 percent fat
- Muscle mass not determined

I failed my test to be a soldier. I was told that 26 percent body fat was the upper limit, so obesity probably saved my life.

I had my first body composition with a bioelectrical impedance scale (four points, two hands and two feet) done at Stormont Obesity Clinic on June 25, 2015, at 63 years old.

- Weight 244.8 pounds
- Waist 43 inches
- Total body fat 31 percent, 75.2 pounds
- Muscle mass 46.1 pounds (but Ohms 486 was low so muscle mass might have been higher)
- Fat-free mass 68.9 percent with 167.4 pounds (lean body weight)

At age 65, I might have developed sarcopenia. As people age, even though their BMI might not change, the skeletal muscle mass decreases as more fat is put on. For men, this is especially true in the legs.

Lean body weight becomes important in the obese for determining medication dosage size, although I suspect it is rarely used for this. Lean body weight needs to be determined to know how many grams of protein per day to eat (2.4 mg/kg lean body weight).

Bioelectrical Impedance Analysis

"BIA is considered reasonably accurate for measuring groups, or for tracking body composition in an individual over a period of time, but is not considered sufficiently accurate for recording of single measurements of individuals. Two-electrode foot-to-foot measurement is less accurate than four-electrode (feet, hands) and eight-electrode measurement."[42]

I am on five diet medications. On March 17, 2017, I increased my liraglutide to 3.0 mg a day. This helped me get down to 200 pounds without changing my diet and walking only twenty to forty minutes a day. I've lost forty pounds since I started Invokana and stopped insulin and Actos. Now the challenge is to maintain weight loss in my reduced obese state as demonstrated in "After *The Biggest Loser*, Their Bodies Fought to Regain Weight," by Gina Kolata.[14]

In 2016 I gained weight, but the obesity clinic at Stormont was pleased with my body composition results. Compare May 16, 2016, when I weighed in at my lowest at 217.3 pounds, to August 17, 2016, at 222.5 pounds. During those two months, I began a high-protein diet (2.4 mg/kg lean body weight) and circuit weight lifting of twenty-five repetitions to preserve muscle mass.[40] My muscle mass increased by 1.8 pounds, body fat decreased by 1.1 percent, fat-free mass increased by 1.2 percent, and body water increased by 1.6 percent.

I did this with an ad libitum Atkins diet. I am never hungry and I drink two to four ounces of alcohol almost every day. This is the bon vivant diet. However, without the benefit of the bioelectric impedance scale, it might look like the five diet medications were failing. I started Qsymia on June 23, 2015, at 244 pounds. At 220 pounds on December 13, 2015, I had lost five pounds of muscle.

CHAPTER 15

Bariatric Surgery: The Last Resort

I went to a conference on obesity in Washington, DC, in October 2015. Dr. Denis Halmi gave a lecture titled "Recidivism after Bariatric Surgery." The most important fact I took away from that lecture on bariatric surgery was that 30 percent of patients regain the lost weight within ten years.[35]

I believe all diet medications should be tried before bariatric surgery is done. The main reason was cited in MedlinePlus on June 6, 2017: "One in five weight loss surgery patients using opioids." This was seven years after the surgery.

To my surprise, new data from Duke University in 2016 claimed the following: "Only 19 of 564 patients undergoing RYGB (3.4%) regained weight back to within an estimated 5% of their baseline weight by 10 years." (Maciejewski, M. et al. "Bariatric Surgery and Long-term Durability of Weight Loss." *JAMA Surgery, 151*(11), 1046–1055. doi10.1001/jamasurg.2016.2317) When I looked at this data more carefully, I found that the study included 1,787 RYGB surgeries. Only nineteen of 564 surgical patients gained most of their weight back after ten years, but what happened to the other 1,223 patients? Sixty-eight percent of patients were lost to follow-up? They probably didn't go back to follow up, because they had regained their weight. If an intention-to-treat analysis was done, the regain number would be much higher. This is the VA, so there must be follow-up data on these surgeries.

More data from the Duke study: "Patients undergoing RYGB lost 21% (95% CI, 11%-31%) more of their baseline weight at 10 years than nonsurgical matches. A total of 405 of 564 patients undergoing RYGB (71.8%) had more than 20% estimated weight loss, and 224 of 564 (39.7%) had more than 30% estimated weight loss at 10 years, compared with 134 of 1247 (10.8%) and 48 of 1247 (3.9%), respectively, of nonsurgical matches."

The usual waterfall results[9] of weight loss studies:

- Nonsurgical patients
- 10.8 percent had more than 20 percent weight loss?
- 3.4 percent had more than 30 percent weight loss?

After fifteen years, there was data regarding sustained weight loss. Again the dropout rate is large, and again there is no explanation.

In a *New York Times* Sunday Review Opinion on September 10, 2016, Dr. Sarah Hallberg and Osama Hamdy write, "It is nonsensical that we're expected to prescribe these (bariatric) techniques to our patients while the medical guidelines don't include another better, safer and far cheaper method: a diet low in carbohydrates."[43]

CHAPTER 16

The First Office Visit Needs Data

Concentrate on preventing arterial plaque and getting type 2 diabetes mellitus patients off insulin and Actos. Obesity comorbidities include type 2 diabetes mellitus, hypertension, hyperlipidemia, cancer, osteoarthritis, cardiovascular disease, obstructive sleep apnea, and asthma. If you have these conditions as a result of obesity, the risks versus benefits of diet medications become apparent. Unfortunately it is more popular to go to bariatric surgery.

First rule: Stop taking medications that make you fat.
Second rule: Out metabolic syndrome.

Check with your physician if you are on medications that cause weight gain and can be replaced with some other drug. For example, replace insulin with Invokana, metformin, and Victoza.

Much of the literature says that most people cannot stay on an Atkins-type diet because stopping carbohydrates is too restrictive. I agree that patients who aren't pre-diabetic and don't have metabolic syndrome might do better on other diets based on individual preference. I went on Atkins many years ago for only one month, and I had the weakness often associated with it. Even now I get leg cramps at bedtime, but the solution is chicken bouillon, magnesium, and perhaps potassium replacement and increased fluid intake. All diets are restrictive. I suspect that failure to give up carbohydrates results from cultural and ethnic conditioning rather than from genetics.

There are no essential carbohydrates, although there are essential fats and amino acids. (Essential means that you'll get sick if you're deficient in them.) Usually after a month, eating fewer carbs is acceptable to most people. No matter which diet the reduced obese choose, they must reduce calories to maintain weight loss, so all diets include restrictions.

LCHF suggests a carbohydrate night, as long as you don't eat a whole pizza, a pint of ice cream, or a pound of pasta. I have found the main benefit of diet medications is that they help me reduce portions and hunger. I've been able to skip my midmorning and midafternoon snacks if I eat 30 grams of protein for both breakfast and lunch. If I need a snack, I stick to a bag of pistachios (1.5 oz, 42 g). After dinner, I relieve my boredom and hunger with a cocktail and a Light and Lively Greek yogurt cup (80 calories).

I ask patients to come to the office fasting so that we can obtain fasting glucose and ketone levels. If the fasting glucose level is 100 or more, then the patient has the first criteria of the metabolic syndrome. At this point the patient needs to start metformin, their first obesity drug, at 500 mg per day.

Update: After reading *Eat Rich, Live Long,* I would also add insulin level to fasting glucose and a two-hour post-prandial glucose to find insulin resistance early.[44]

One quarter of the USA population has metabolic syndrome, according to *Current Medical Diagnosis and Treatment 2017* (p. 12). Metabolic syndrome is defined as having three or more of the following: fasting glucose greater than 110, triglycerides greater than 150, hypertension, HDLc less than 40 for men and less than 50 for women, and abdominal obesity.

I use the NCEP ATP 3 criteria from 2005 to diagnose metabolic syndrome. The main difference is that the fasting glucose is 100 or greater. The measurement of the waist is done at the level of the iliac crest: >40 inches or 102 cm for men, >35 inches or 88 cm for women. Measurements for Asians are >89 cm for men and >79 cm for women. Also, if the triglyceride/HDLc ratio is 3:1 or greater, I will consider the patient as having metabolic syndrome.

Insulin resistance impairs the capacity of the insulin receptor to signal the fat cell to halt triglyceride breakdown by lipase and increases glucose uptake by glucose transport proteins. This increases the release of fatty acids into central circulation and decreases uptake of glucose by fat cells.

I advise patients to use any diet that has worked for them in the past. A low-carb diet might not work as well for someone who doesn't have pre-diabetes, metabolic syndrome, or type 2 diabetes mellitus. However, I would still suggest that these patients switch to a low-carb diet when they hit the plateau, so that they'll go into nutritional ketoacidosis, which may help with their low leptin causing increased hunger.

Eating ad libitum—high protein, five times a day—will help minimize hunger. Nevertheless, the sponge syndrome will eventually cause you to begin regaining weight. That's the time to begin taking diet medications to maintain weight loss. If you're already on diet meds, consider adding another one if you continue to gain weight.

PART 2

The Tubby Theory and Cardiovascular Disease

CHAPTER 17

Risk for Heart Attack

The next step in the office visit is to determine your risk for a cardiovascular event such as a stroke or heart attack. This is done with a pooled-cohort risk assessment that predicts your ten-year risk for a first atherosclerotic cardiovascular disease (ASCVD) event

At 119, my total cholesterol is too low for this calculator, so I was forced to use a higher number is get an evaluation. This probably represents me since my mine is treated and my glucose Hg A1C is usually 7.0 or lower.

I advise patients to get more data. Find out if you have atherosclerotic plaque, for example, which will change your risk up or down. Get a coronary artery calcium (CAC), CT calcium score ($50), and a carotid intimal media thickness (CIMT) ultrasound ($100).

If you have plaque or atheroma, then you have the disease of atherosclerosis and it increases your risk of an event. If your CAC is zero, that decreases your risk considerably. If you are symptomatic_and your CAC is zero, you still have a 16 percent risk.

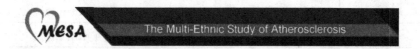

MESA 10-Year CHD Risk with Coronary Artery Calcification

Above link says, "The estimated 10 year risk of a CHD event for a person with this risk factor profile including coronary calcium is 12.5 percent. The estimated ten-year risk of a CHD event for a person with this risk factor profile if we did not factor in their coronary calcium score would be 11.1 percent.

144 126

CAC is not advised on a routine follow-up basis, because statin treatment will cause an increase in the CAC number.

CHAPTER 18

CIMT and CAC: High-Fat Diet Did Not Equal "Clogged Arteries"

Does a diet that is 60 percent fat, including so-called bad and good fats, cause atherosclerosis? That's the big question about the Atkins diet. I documented my CIMT from 2009 to 2017 while on an Atkins diet, and my results were good.

CIMTs at KUMC in Dr. Moriarty's Lipo-apheresis clinic:

Average CCA Mean Average CCA Max Region

12-17-09	0.599 mm	0.741 mm
12-8-11	0.563 mm less	0.661 mm less
12-20-12	0.566 mm more	0.676 mm more
12-19-13	0.583 mm more	0.709 mm more
11-20-14	0.575 mm less	0.679 mm less
12-03-15	0.555 mm less	0.675 mm less
12-08-16	0.611 mm more	0.74 mm more
12-14-17	0.570 mm less	0.671 mm less

CAC reports below over ten years:

	Calcium score	Calcium volume
2-6-01	8.93	8.02
1-10-06	20.5	57.5
12-9-11	7.9	5.9
7-21-16	144	126

Over eight years, I have had regression. More importantly, I have not had the progression that a 66-year-old, type 2 diabetic might be expected to have over eight years on an Atkins diet with 60 percent fat.

There will be natural thickening of the intimal wall with aging as well. My CAC increased from 7.9 to 144, but this is a well-known phenomenon that occurs when intensive statin therapy is used. However, my increase in calcium score is compensated for by an increase in my CAC volume, not by a true increase in plaque. This is a good reason not to bother with follow-up CAC scans too often.

I received a critique from another Fellow of the National Lipid Association. I told him that a 0.034 mm change is significant according to the Neil Stone lipid manual. My friend wrote to Thomas Barringer, a national expert on CIMT. Dr. Barringer's reply basically validated my opinion because he agreed with everything about which my friend had critiqued me. According to Barringer, IMT progression has shown no association with subsequent cardiovascular events except in the IMPROVE study (Baldassare, et al.). In 2013, the published results of that study showed that an entirely new IMT variable—the IMT segment showing the fastest increase in maximum dimension—was associated with an increase in CVEs. I do not use CIMTs for determining cardiovascular risk.

My purpose was to determine if I would lay on substantial plaque in carotids because of being on a Atkins diet at 60 percent fat. Most of the fat was in beef, eggs, bacon, butter, and mayonnaise—or the so-called "good" fats of the Mediterranean diet.

CHAPTER 19

What Is the Best Cholesterol Test?

In my opinion, the best test is the liposcience LDLp done by nuclear magnetic resonance. The second best is the non-HDL cholesterol test because it's the cheapest. The third is the apoB test done by immune assay technique.

The new view is to determine the number of cholesterol remnants on your lab test. The formula is to subtract LDLc and HDLc from total cholesterol. The result is the amount of cholesterol remnants. For example, my total cholesterol (115) minus my LDLc (57) equals 58. When I then subtract my HDLc (48), my total cholesterol remnants equals 10. (Greater than 30 is considered high.)

Physicians need to stop following a patient's LDLc and switch to non-HDLc, at the very least. There is too much discordance between LDLc and LDLp,[45] especially in patients with metabolic syndrome, diabetes type 2, or a high triglyceride level.

Official guidelines for LDLp and apoB seem a little high to me. In *The Tubby Theory from Topeka*, I advised that non-HDLc be called the Tubby Factor. It is easier to remember to ask your doctor, "What's my Tubby Factor?" Non-HDLc is more accurate in predicting future risk than LDLc.

More accurate than both of those is the particle number. (Don't get bogged down with particle size, HDLc, or triglycerides.) ApoB and LDLp are the best tests. The LDLp ion method done by Quest lab does not use the numbers in this chart.

These are the American Association of Clinical Endocrinologists (AACE) lipid targets for patients with type 2 diabetes and one major ASCVD or established ASCVD: LDLc <70, non-HDL <100, triglycerides <150, Apo B (particles) <80, and LDLp (particles) <1,000. Major risk factors include a family history of ASCVD, high blood pressure, low HDLc, and smoking. (Garber, A., et al. "Consensus Statement by the American Association of Clinical Endocrinologists and American College of Endocrinology on the Comprehensive Type 2 Diabetes Management Algorithm: 2018 Executive Summary." *Endocrine Practice, 24*(1), 91–120. doi:10.4158/CS-2017-0153)

Here are the AACE recommended LDLc targets for 2018[46]: high risk <100, very high risk <70, and extreme risk <55. The non-HDLc targets are high risk <130, very high risk <100, and extreme risk <80.

One way to know if you have atherosclerotic disease is to get a CAC and CIMT. Guidelines do advise using these studies for further clarification of risk.

With the publication of studies such as IMPROVE-IT and HPS2-THRIVE, cholesterol guidelines say that nonstatin therapies may be considered in patients who respond poorly to statins or cannot tolerate optimal doses of them. Non-statin therapy options include (1) referral to a lipid specialist and a registered dietitian nutritionist, (2) ezetimibe (Zetia, Merck), (3) bile acid sequestrants, and (4) PCSK9 inhibitors such as alirocumab (Praluent, Sanofi/Regeneron) and evolocumab (Repatha, Amgen). (5) Mipomersen (Kynamro, Isis Pharmaceutical/Genzyme), lomitapide (Juxtapid, Aegerion) and (6) LDL apheresis may be considered by lipid specialists for patients with familial hypercholesterolemia, according to Lloyd-Jones and colleagues.[47]

It is outrageous that niacin was removed from the nonstatin therapy options. This removal of niacin is based on an inaccurate analysis of IMPROVE-IT and HPS2-THRIVE.[33]

Dr. Sniderman, one of the best lipidologists, explains how he approaches the problem of treatment with statins and nonstatins:

> The first thing I do is measure apoB to determine whether treatment is necessary or not. If apoB is elevated, then all things being equal, treatment needs to be seriously considered. Treatment is a collaborative process between the patient and the physician and involves diet, exercise, and lifestyle as well as pharmacologic agents if indicated. For the majority, my target for LDL-lowering therapy is an apoB <75 mg/dL. For those at very high risk, my target is an apoB <65 mg/dL. These are the equivalent population levels to the LDL-C and non-HDL-C targets chosen by many recent guideline groups. The apoB targets chosen by many of the guideline groups are much too high. It seems that once one group selected values, the others just repeated them.[48]

Thus according to this last CIMT, I have not had regression, but I also haven't had the progression that a 65-year-old diabetic type 2 might expect over seven years. There will be natural thickening of the intimal wall with aging. Likewise my CAC increased from 7.9 to 144, but this is a well-known phenomenon that occurs when intensive statin therapy is used. This is a good reason not to bother with follow-up CAC scans.

In 2009, I tried to get high-risk patients to the following goals:[5]

- Tubby Factor (non-HDLc) less than 80. Inexpensive test.
- LDLc less than 70 usually calculated and inaccurate in insulin resistance
- Apo B less than 60 (immunoassay) particle count
- LDLp less than 750 (done by Liposcience NMR) particle count. Best test, in my opinion.

The 2014 American Diabetic guidelines are still using the old LDLc numbers. Diabetics often have discordance between LDLc, Tubby Factor, and particle number.

The National Lipid Association now uses non-HDL cholesterol as an official target. I predicted this in my book in 2009. LDLp and apoB are still not an official target of any group.[50]

Contrary to the ACC/AHA guidelines, the NLA guidelines say that nonstatin therapy should be considered in patients who can't tolerate statin therapy or high-dose statin therapy. Nonstatin therapy medications by a second or third agent may be considered for patients who have not reached goals for atherogenic cholesterol levels.

CHAPTER 20

Tubby Theory from Topeka Update

From my book *The Tubby Theory from Topeka*,[5] published in January 2010: "The *Tubby Theory* is that we can prevent heart disease with simvastatin/Endur-Acin in America for less than $100 a year if we find the subclinical atherosclerosis *early* with CAC/CIMT" (p. 9). I wrote this in December 2009, eight years ago.

Cardiologists did not know what a non-HDL cholesterol was. The ignored number in the life of Tim Russert, the moderator on NBC's *Meet the Press*, and his post-mortem analysis was his non-HDL cholesterol. Apparently no one asked a lipidologist. Last month I learned that remnant particles should be calculated as well.

Total cholesterol minus HDLc = non-HDLc (Tubby Factor)
Total cholesterol minus HDLc minus LDLc = remnant cholesterol

Here's Tim Russert's updated risk:
Total cholesterol (155) minus HDLc (37) minus LDLc (68) = 50 remnants
His remnants were abnormally high; normal is less than 30.

The Tubby Theory has held up well. Many experts, such as Robinson and Sniderman, now believe that treating early will improve outcomes.[57] CAC and CIMT are tools to persuade the nonsymptomatic patient to start statins early, although it is a mistake to go to a high-dose statin too soon. Here's the triple therapy that I recommended in 2009:

1. Start with the lowest statin dose.
2. Check non-HDLc in one month. If not at goal, switch from statin to 1,000 mg of Endur-Acin, an over-the-counter niacin with a proprietary wax matrix formula.
3. Check non-HDL in one month. If not at goal, switch to ezetimibe (Zetia). Sometimes half a tablet is sufficient.

Eight years after I published *The Tubby Theory from Topeka*, a friend said to me, "You have been talking about coronary calcium scores for a long time. Were you ahead of your colleagues or in step with them?" I wrote that book after I passed the lipid boards and Tim Russert died. No one in NLA had spoken to the national media about Russert's non-HDLc not being treated to goal, probably because they were afraid of being sued. I thus wrote a book about treating patients in my practice aggressively, using the teachings of my mentors at NLA and quoting them throughout the book.

I called non-HDLc the Tubby Factor because neither patients nor physicians could remember "non-HDL cholesterol" or how to calculate it. Non-HDLc is usually discordant with LDLc in patients with metabolic syndrome, and 80 percent of these patients are obese, usually with central obesity.

Since my book in 2010, I have been gratified to see that CAC and CIMT have proven themselves as significant and independent risk predictors for CVD. AHA/ACA guidelines in 2013 by Stone[49] use CAC or CIMT in low-risk patients to determine whether statins should be started.

Niacin is under attack as being a dangerous drug, which I believe is just silly.[33] If low-dose wax-matrix niacin (over-the-counter Endur-Acin) 1,000 mg/d is used with low-dose Lipitor 20 mg/d early[57] in the disease of subclinical atherosclerosis for long-term treatment, I believe we can prevent most CVD. Some patients will need Zetia (now available in its generic form, ezetimibe.)

I am proud of *The Tubby Theory from Topeka*. Even the low-fat diet I suggested might be suitable for some folks who are insulin sensitive and hyper-absorbers of cholesterol. Atkins doesn't work for everyone. In the present obesity epidemic, I think that most obese have pre-diabetes, metabolic syndrome, or insulin resistance. An Atkins-type diet is best for these people.

My experience with being on a 60 percent Atkins diet since 2011 did not increase my atheroma on CIMT or CAC.[58] People should use the diet that has previously worked for them. For lifelong maintenance of weight loss, I advise switching to Atkins because you can eat ad libitum and test yourself for nutritional ketosis. Most reduced obese will ultimately need diet medication to avoid the terrible hunger that low leptin[34] will cause after years of dieting.

There was an article by Denise Grady in the *New York Times* about Tim Russert's death.[52] My response to Grady's article is that yes, we could pinpoint Russert's higher risk at that time, but he needed to have his non-HDL cholesterol calculated. Grady's article doesn't mention Glagov remodeling of the arteries, which is why a nuclear stress test was false negative on Mr. Russert one month before his death. To my knowledge, I'm the only one who wrote about this in 2009.

In a metabolic patient such as Mr. Russert, there is usually discordance between LDLc and LDLp or non-HDLc. Mr. Russert was thought to have normal LDLc, but with his high triglycerides, this was unlikely. When his non-HDLc was found to be high, the LDLp or apo B particle test should have been done. Then those numbers could have been treated to goal with medication.

In 2009, I advised my patients get their LDLp below 750, their Apo B below 60, and their non-HDL cholesterol below 80. If they had plaque on their CAC or CIMT, they needed to reverse that plaque.

In May 2008, Tim Russert's non-HDL cholesterol was 118 (TC 155 - HDLC 37). He was clearly not treated to goal with the information at hand. There is even discordance with non-HDLc and particle numbers. A $100 blood test for the particle number should be obtained before a $1,000 invasive angiogram. Some doctors say that people like Mr. Russert, with no symptoms but risk factors such as a thickened heart, should have an angiogram, in which a catheter is threaded into the coronary arteries, dye is injected, and X-rays are taken to look for blockages.

Again this is a picture of the lumen of the artery. Very likely, most of Mr. Russert's disease was in the wall of the artery, only to be seen by IVUS. However, a CIMT could give us an idea about what might be going on in the wall of the coronary artery, if the carotid wall was much thicker than it should be. In my practice, I've had eleven patients with negative CAC but positive CIMT; they complement each other.

That same *New York Times* article says that statins reduce risk only by 70 percent, leaving a residual risk of 30 percent. Here's my response:

- The multiplier effect[57] should be used to treat the other residual risk of 30 percent.
- Find the plaque early with CAC and CIMT.
- Treat early and for a long time with low-dose combination therapy.
- Take a low dose to avoid side effects in the long term.
- Keep LDLp below 750 to 1,000

This is what I said in the *Tubby Theory* in 2009, and I showed the results of doing it in my practice in my book.[61]

I wrote *The Tubby Theory from Topeka*[5] to alert people that Tim Russert's death could have been prevented if the discordance between LDLc and non-HDL-cholesterol had been recognized. Better data with LDL particle numbers should have been obtained. Now with PCSK9 we know that LDLc levels of 39 mg/dl are therapeutic and reduce plaque as determined by IVUS (intravascular ultrasound).

"Treatment with statins plus evolocumab achieved mean LDL-C levels of 36.6 mg/dL, produced atheroma regression with a mean change in percent of atheroma volume of about 1% ($P < .001$), and induced regression in a greater percentage of patients. The clinical benefits of LDL-C as low as 20 mg/dL shown in this trial warrant further investigation."[60]

CHAPTER 21

Niacin Is Still a Great Drug[33]

Should guidelines for drugs be established without head-to-head trials? "In the absence of high quality head-to-head drug comparison trials to determine the relative efficacy of the individual drugs, choice of therapy should be based upon efficacy, safety, cost, convenience, and other patient-related factors." This comes from *Up to Date* on choosing drugs for osteoporosis.

Consensus Committee, April 6, 2016 "ACC Expert Consensus Decision Pathway on the Role of Non-Statin Therapies for LDL-Cholesterol Lowering in the Management of Atherosclerotic Cardiovascular Disease Risk." My rebuttals are enclosed in brackets.

"The value of patient-provider interaction in clinical decision making when non-statin therapies are considered:

1. examining the extent of available scientific evidence for net clinical benefit,
    [Decades of trials show the benefit of niacin.]
2. safety,
    [Serious side effects associated with high doses 2,000 mg or greater or not significant in AIM-HIGH (infection and stroke).]
3. tolerability,
    [The wax matrix preparation of Endur-Acin does not have the flushing effect, especially at 1,000 mg a day.]
4. potential for drug-drug interactions,
    [Wine may increase the flush, so don't take with nicotine.]
5. efficacy of additional LDL-C lowering,
    [See Guyton's list of trials below.]
6. cost,
    [Endur-Acin is less than $100 for one thousand 500 mg tablets.]
7. convenience,
    [Order on internet and take two 500 mg tablets at breakfast or lunch. Insert says to take the two doses separately, but I have taken 1,000 mg at a time for twenty years.]
8. medication storage,
    [No refrigeration needed.]
9. pill burden,
    [Only two pills a day.]

10. route of administration,
    [Oral.]
11. and patient preference."
    [Most patients want the least expensive medicine and don't want needles.]

From a 2009 article in the *New England Journal of Medicine* on a head-to-head comparison of niacin and Zetia (ezetimibe):[62] "As compared with ezetimibe, niacin had greater efficacy regarding the change in mean carotid intima-media thickness over 14 months (P = 0.003), leading to significant reduction of both mean (P = 0.001) and maximal carotid intima-media thickness. Paradoxically, greater reductions in the LDL cholesterol level in association with ezetimibe were significantly associated with an increase in the carotid intima-media thickness."

Niacin was the first lipid-lowering drug to improve mortality in the Coronary Drug Project,[63] in which "Mortality in the niacin group was 11% lower than in the placebo group (52.0 versus 58.2%; p = 0.0004)" after fifteen years. This was not a blind, random-controlled study. Yet somehow niacin failed to make the list of nonstatin drugs allowed on the list. PCSK9, which costs $1,000 per month, had new trials in 2017 and 2018.

Glagov 2017: "Clinical benefits of LDL-C as low as 20 mg/dL shown."[60]

Fournier 2018: "Patients closer to their most recent MI, with multiple prior MIs, or with residual multivessel CAD are at high risk for major vascular events and experience substantial risk reductions with LDL-C lowering with evolocumab."[64]

Odyssey 2018: "In individuals with T2DM and mixed dyslipidaemia on maximally tolerated statin, alirocumab showed superiority to UC in non-HDL cholesterol reduction and was generally well tolerated."[65]

Odyssey 2018: "15% reduction in major adverse coronary event (MACE) p = 0.0003. 29% mortality reduction for LDLc > 99 mg/dl."[66]

In 2018, the American Association of Clinical Endocrinologists created a new category of extreme risk. The LDLc target goal for these people was < 55.[66]

Reference from Table 26.2 from J. R. Guyton et al.

List of randomized niacin trials with clinical cardiovascular outcomes:

1. HATS: clinical events reduced by 70%
2. AFREGS: clinical events reduced by 50%
3. CLAS: more overall regression of plaque (p < 0.002)
4. UCSF-SCOR: coronary angio regression (p < 0.039)
5. FATS: regression of plaque and 73% reduced clinical events (P < 0.05)
6. HARP: no change in coronary angiographic progression

7. ARBITER 2-3: mean regression of CIMT at 2 years (p < 0.001)
8. THOENES CIMT: mean regression of CIMT (p = 0.021)
9. ARBITER-6 HALTS: reduction CIMT (p < 0.001)
10. CAROTID MRI: reduction in carotid wall area by MRI (p = 0.03)

Niacin was dropped from the guidelines because AIM-HIGH and HPS-THRIVE were stopped early. These were not LDLc-lowering trials; LDLc was already at goal with statins. These were HDLc and triglyceride trials. The guidelines don't have targets for HDLc and advise triglycerides less than 500. Many trials have proven the validity of the hypothesis: the lower the LDLc, the better. The major goal is to lower LDLc. Niacin decreased LDLc levels after year three of the AIM HIGH trial. Why, then, was niacin dropped from the guidelines?

Concerning the IMPROVE-IT trial with Zetia: "It took 7 years of follow-up for us to reach that many events, so some investigators were wondering if this would be the eternal trial," Cannon said. "But that was really good news because it meant that the treatment was working: we were actually doing good for our patients." It should, however, be noted that 42 percent of patients, regardless of treatment, stopped the study drug before the end of the trial. Zetia was added to the list by the consensus committee because it had the IMPROVE-IT positive outcome.

If AIM-HIGH with niacin had gone out to seven years, it might also have had a positive outcome for niacin. However, there were some illnesses in patients on niacin, so AIM-HIGH, a government study, was stopped early. Later those illnesses were found not to be statistically significant, but I believe that's why the committee left niacin off the list of advised drugs.

At the Philadelphia NLA meeting on May 20, 2017, several speakers said they don't use niacin anymore because of "toxic" side effects from niacin in AIM HIGH and HPS- THRIVE. However, there are other opinions: "Recent results published by the two large clinical studies, AIM-HIGH and HPS-THRIVE, have led to the impugnation of niacin's role in future clinical practice. However, due to several methodological flaws in the AIM-HIGH and HPS2-THRIVE studies, the pleiotrophic effects of niacin now deserve thorough evaluation."

Last year at the NLA master's program, a slide bullet said, "Significant excesses of serious adverse events (SAEs) due to known and unrecognized side-effects of niacin. Over 4 years, ER niacin/laropiprant caused SAEs in approximately 30 patients per 1,000." Was this caused by niacin or lapopirant?

Specifically in HPS2-THRIVE:

- coronary death placebo had 0.1% less 302 versus 291 p 0.63
- hemorrhagic stroke placebo had 0.2% less 114 versus 89 p 0.08

These are not significant differences. "If the p-value is less than 0.05, we reject the null hypothesis that there's no difference between the means and conclude that a significant difference does exist."

Slide on effect of ERN/LRPT on serious adverse events with significant p:

- Diabetic complication 3.7%
- New onset diabetes 1.8%
- Infection 1.4%
- Gastrointestinal 1.0%

The problem with these SAEs with a significant p is that we don't know what's responsible, niacin or LRPT.

What I find difficult to understand is why niacin's legacy effect has been ignored. It has decades of efficacy and safety, and it's inexpensive. PCSK9 is expensive, but it can get LDLc down to 39 or lower. Patients at high risk who can't take statins need this. The AACE guidelines now have an extreme risk level and advise getting the LDLc > 55.[67]

The Tubby Theory alternative is to take the lowest dose of a statin plus Endur-Acin (over-the-counter niacin), 1,000 mg plus Zetia (ezetimibe) one-half tablet. This combination needs to be attempted before using the very expensive PCSK9 drug. The lower doses have fewer side effects, and the three drugs are very likely to get to goal, as I showed in my list of patients in my book from 2010. The doctor can increase the statin slowly each month to maximum dosage and increase Zetia to a full tablet while monitoring for side effects. If this sequential step plan of triple therapy does not work, then of course go to PCSK9.

Since I wrote *The Tubby Theory from Topeka*, the data has confirmed the premise that the lower the LDLc, the better. Now we don't know a normal level of LDLc. The target LDLc depends on the patient's amount of risk. Thus most believe it is not the pleiotrophic effects or the raising of HDLc that improves treatment—it's how low you can get the patient's LDLc.

Many people might believe the pill burden to be too great, especially if four daily tabs of Lovaza (fish oil) are ordered to lower triglycerides. When I practiced infectious disease, I learned that HIV patients will take a huge number of pills to save their lives. Compliance was often determined with frequent HIV virus count checks. In statin therapy, compliance can also be checked with LDLp and a triglyceride check every three to four months.

I strongly believe the big problem of side effects with statins is caused by starting at too high a dose. At a low dose (1,000 mg) of niacin, it is unlikely that the bad side effects seen in AIM HIGH and HPS-THRIVE will occur.

Zeta has finally had a positive outcome trial (IMPROVE-IT), right at the time of ezetimibe, the generic version, becoming available.

If we truly want to prevent atherosclerotic heart disease, we need to treat people earlier and for life to keep their LDLp under 750 or 1,000 or apo B around 60. This is the multiplier effect.[57] A complex plaque that has been present for a long time will unlikely be cured with medications. This is the 30 percent residual risk. However we need to treat early to prevent the simple plaque from becoming complex. Thus the legacy safety and price and efficacy call for the option of triple therapy before injecting PCSK9, which is expensive and does not have the decades of legacy safety or efficacy that niacin has.

CHAPTER 22

The Multiplier Effect[57]

The Tubby Theory treats patients very early in their disease of elevated non-HDL cholesterol (Tubby Factor) with a CAC score of one or greater or other major risk factors. Even if the risk calculator is less than 10 percent over ten years (5 to 10 percent), I recommend statin therapy if atherosclerosis is present on CAC or CIMT. Any amount of plaque or atheroma is potentially deadly, and the progression of plaque can be stopped with a low LDLp < 1,000 or non-HDLc level < 100. I also advise getting the LDLp < 750 or non-HDLc level < 80 to get regression of plaque.

In 2010 this was considered an aggressive approach, but it has become much more acceptable. In 2018, PCSK9 trials (Fournier and Odyssey) have gotten LDLc below 40 with no ill effects.

June 28, 2016
Update on the multiplier effect using statins early in treating CVD

I've been touting my multiplier effect theory since I described using it in my lipidology practice in my 2010 book, *The Tubby Theory from Topeka*. In a *JAMA* research letter on May 18, 2016, Dr. Allan Sniderman writes, "Our findings highlight the need to refine strategies to identify individuals younger than 60 years who are candidates for preventive therapies. Several options exist. The risk threshold used by the lipid guidelines could be lowered to the optional 5 percent level, age and sex specific thresholds could be adopted, or additional risk factors might be added."

In 2009 in Topeka, I was getting non-HDLc, LDLp, CAC, and CIMT on my patients. As with other models in treating chronic diseases such as hypertension, HIV, and diabetes, multiple drugs are used for more efficacy (synergy) and at lower doses to minimize the side effects for lifelong therapy.

The same is true to lower LDLp, apoB, or non-HDLc. Before 2009, I prescribed a triple low-dose therapy with simvastatin, niacin, and Zetia (ezetimibe) for less than $100 a year. In 2018 we have generic ezetimibe (Zetia), generic atorvastatin (Lipitor) is available at a low price, and generic rosuvastatin (Crestor) is also available and will be at a lower price. My niacin of choice is an over-the-counter wax matrix preparation called Endur-Acin at 1,000 mg a day. One thousand 500 mg pills purchased on the internet costs less than $100. The multiplier effect of combining these drugs and prescribing them early, before complex plaque lesions occur, ideally will reduce the 30 percent residual risk considerably.

The new drug is PCSK9, which is expensive, but the recent Fourier and Odyssey trials showed no serious side effects with LDLc of 30. The lower LDLc showed 15 percent fewer cardiovascular events in statin plus PCS9K arm versus statin alone control arm.

These trials continue to validate that lower is better with LDLc.

Endnotes

1 Ludwig, David. (2016). *Always Hungry.*

2 Aronne, Louis J. (2016). *The Change Your Biology Diet.*

3 The Look AHEAD Research Group. (2013). "Cardiovascular Effects of Intensive Lifestyle Intervention in Type 2 Diabetes." *New England Journal of Medicine, 369*, 145–154. doi:10.1056/NEJMoa1212914

4 Tucker, Todd. (2008). *The Great Starvation Experiment: The Heroic Men Who Starved So That Millions Could Live.*

5 Edwards, Brian Scott. (2010). *The Tubby Theory from Topeka.*

6 Jacobson, T. et al. "National Lipid Association Recommendations for Patient-Centered Management of Dyslipidemia: Part 1—Full Report." *Journal of Clinical Lipidology, 9*(2), 129–169.

7 Edwards, Brian Scott. *The Tubby Traveler from Topeka.*

8 PCSK9 guidelines (2017).

9 Waterfall results on my blog site. First taught to me by Dr. Gardner concerning his ATOZ trial.

10 Look AHEAD trial.

11 Livingston, Edward H. (2018). "Reimagining Obesity in 2018." *JAMA* 319(3), 238–240. doi:10.1001/jama.2017.21779.

"Six years ago, when *JAMA* last published a theme issue on obesity, there was optimism that progress was being made in preventing and treating obesity. As time has passed, so too has the optimism, as reports continued to show that the prevalence of obesity was increasing and, most important, rapidly increasing in children. A year and a half ago, there was a call to reconsider obesity and view it in new ways with the hope of better managing this very consequential clinical problem. In response, *JAMA* has revisited obesity in the form of a theme issue."

12 Cruise, Jorge. *The 3-Hour Diet.*

13 Rudolph L. Leibel, M.D. The man cheated of the Nobel Prize.

14 Kolata, Gina. (2 May, 2016). "After *The Biggest Loser,* Their Bodies Fought to Regain Weight." *New York Times.*

15 Gretchen Reynolds. (2016). *New York Times.*

16 The Set Point video on Fat Nation.

17   Dr. Rosenbaum explains leptin.

18   Low-carbohydrate, high-fat diets of different degrees:

- Westman, E., Phinney, S., & Volek, J. (2010). *The New Atkins for a New You: The Ultimate Diet for Shedding Weight and Feeling Great.*
- Ludwig, D. *Always Hungry? Conquer Cravings, Retrain Your Fat Cells, and Lose Weight Permanently.*
- Aronne, L. *The Change Your Biology Diet: The Proven Program for Lifelong Weight Loss.*
- Agatston, A. *The South Beach Diet: The Delicious, Doctor-Designed, Foolproof Plan for Fast and Healthy Weight Loss.*
- Cohen, I. *Dr. Cohen's New Hippocratic Diet Guide.*

19   Greenway, Frank. (2015). "Physiological Adaptations to Weight Loss and Factors Favouring Weight Regain." *International Journal of Obesity, 39*, 1188–1196. doi:10.1038/ijo.2015.59

20   Kolata, Gina. (2007). *Rethinking Thin: The New Science of Weight Loss—and the Myths and Realities of Dieting.*

21   Vogt, M. C., & Brüning, J. C. (2013). "CNS Insulin Signaling in the Control of Energy Homeostatis and Glucose Metabolism: From Embryo to Old Age." *Trends in Endocrinology and Metabolism, 24*(2), 76–84. doi:10.1016/j.tem.2012.11.004

22   Ochner et al. article. (February 11, 2015).

23   *Scientific American* article on global warming.

24   *Clinical Nutrition.* (January 2016).

25   *Journal of Applied Physiology.* (July 2016).

26   Documented by bioelectrical impedance scale.

27   Second Gretchen Reynolds article from *New York Times.*

28   Hopkin, Michael. (2008). "Fat Cell Numbers Stay Constant Through Adult Life." *Nature.* doi:10.1038/news.2008.800

29   MiRNA exomes from fat cells.

30   I suggest a protein drink between meals for a snack or a replacement meal such as the following:

- Protein Premier (30g protein, 160 calories, 3g fat) replacement meal
- EAS MYO (42g protein, 300 calories, 7g fat) replacement meal for intense weight lifters.

Premier Protein Clear Protein Drink (20g protein, 90 calories, no sugar). I add this snack to Powerade Zero Fruit Punch to cut the sweetness.

- **Atkins shake** (15g protein, 160 calories, 9g fat) snack

31   National Weight Control Registry. (2011).

32 Edwards, Brian S. (April 21, 2018). "The Tubby Factor Explained." *The Tubby Traveler from Topeka*. http://meandgin.blogspot.com/2018/04/the-tubby-factor-explained.html

33 Niacin articles.

34 Sponge syndrome.

35 Bariatric surgery. *JAMA, 303*(11), 1122–1131. (2012).

36 Sumithran, Priya, et al. (2011). "Long-Term Persistence of Hormonal Adaptations to Weight Loss." *New England Journal of Medicine, 365*, 1597–1604. doi:10.1056/NEJMoa1105816

37 Parlee, S., Lentz, S., Mori, H., & MacDougald, O. (2014). "Quantifying Size and Number of Adipocytes in Adipose Tissue." *Methods Enzymol, 537*, 93–122.

38 Wagner et al. "Hypodopaminergic Reward Deficit Syndrome." (p. 7).

Also: Blum, K., Thanos, P., & Gold, M. (2014). "Dopamine and Glucose, Obesity, and Reward Deficiency Syndrome." *Frontiers in Psychology, 5*, 919. doi:10.3389/fpsyg.2014.00919

39 David Ludwig, Summary of an Expert Roundtable on the Role of 100% Fruit Juice.

40 Into the breach of weight loss and muscle loss.

41 Look AHEAD results. (2014). *New England Journal of Medicine.*

42 Bioelectrical impedance analysis (BIA).

43 McKenzie, A., et al. (2017). "A Novel Intervention Including Individualized Nutritional Recommendations Reduces Hemoglobin A1c Level, Medication Use, and Weight in Type 2 Diabetes." *JMIR Diabetes, 2*(1), e5. doi:10.2196/diabetes.6981

"Conclusions: These initial results indicate that an individualized program delivered and supported remotely that incorporates nutritional ketosis can be highly effective in improving glycemic control and weight loss in adults with T2D while significantly decreasing medication use."

44 Cummins, Ivor, & Gerber, Jeffry. (2018). *Eat Rich, Live Long: Mastering the Low-Carb & Keto Spectrum for Weight Loss and Longevity.*

45 Discordance documented in *Tubby Theory from Topeka* patient data.

46 AACE guidelines (2018).

47 JACC guidelines (2016).

48 Interview Dr. Sniderman in Round Table.

49 ACC/AHA guidelines (2013). Neil Stone, MD.

50   Non-HDLc guidelines by NLA (2017 update).

51   Ebling *JAMA* article on reduced thermogenesis (2012). "Among overweight and obese young adults compared with pre-weight loss energy expenditure, isocaloric feeding following 10–15% weight loss resulted in decreases in REE and TEE that were greatest with the low fat diet, intermediate with the low glycemic index diet, and least with the very low CHO diet."

52   Grady, Denise. (June 24, 2008). "From a Prominent Death, Some Painful Truths." *New York Times*.

53   Friedman, Jeffrey. (2016). "The Long Road to Leptin." *Journal of Clinical Investigation, 126*(12), 4727–4734. doi:10.1172/JCI91578

54   Farr, O., Gavrieli, A., & Mantzoros, C. (2015). "Leptin Applications in 2015: What Have We Learned About Leptin and Obesity?" *Current Opinion in Endocrinology, Diabetes, and Obesity, 22*(5), 353–359. doi:10.1097/MED.0000000000000184

55   MacLean, P., Higgins, J., Giles, E., Sherk, V., & Jackman, M. (2015). "The Role for Adipose Tissue in Weight Regain After Weight Loss." *Obesity Review, 16*, 45–54. doi:10.1111/obr.12255

56   Flier, J., & Maratos-Flier, E. (2017). "Leptin's Physiologic Role: Does the Emperor of Energy Balance Have No Clothes?" *Cell Metabolism, 26*(1), 24–26. doi:10.1016/j.cmet.2017.05.013

57   Multiplier effect.

58   My poster presented at NLA NOLA meeting.

59   Consensus Committee (April 6, 2016).

60   Glagov trial (December 2017).

61   The clinical data of my lipid clinic (2009).

62   Niacin vs. Zetia (ezetimibe); head-to-head trial. (2009). *New England Journal of Medicine, 361*, 2113–2122.

63   Coronary Drug Project, fifteen-year results.

64   Fourier trial (2018).

65   The Odyssey Dm-Dyslipidemia randomized trial.

66   Pocock, S., & Collier, T. (2018). "Critical Appraisal of the 2018 ACC Scientific Sessions Late-Breaking Trials From a Statistician's Perspective." *Journal of the American College of Cardiology*. doi:10.1016/j.jacc.2018.04.015

67   AACE guidelines (2018).

Epilogue

The main message of this book is that the sponge syndrome will cause a person to regain weight despite Atkins because the low leptin levels tell their brain that they're starving, and the brain will use compensatory hormonal pathways to force a reduced obese patient to gain weight. Based on my personal experience with chronic obesity, I believe that the only way to maintain weight for longer than ten years with satiety is with multiple diet medications.

The major challenges to the treatment of chronic obesity include the high cost of diet medications and the need to stay on diet medications and a restrictive diet for the rest of your life. Some people are offered bariatric surgery rather than trying an LCHF diet with nutritional ketosis. Physicians must learn about diet medications and use them as a first drug, especially if the patient is on insulin, rather than as a last resort.

Don't ever tell a reduced obese patient that they regained weight because they didn't exercise enough (60 to 90 minutes per day) or stick to a starvation diet (1,500 calories per day), despite this being the present guideline to maintain weight loss. Ask your physician if he or she has read Gina Kolata's article "After *The Biggest Lose*r, Their Bodies Fought to Regain Weight" *(New York Times*, May 2, 2016).

It's all about never losing your fat cells. When adipocytes are shrunken in the reduced obese, they are low in leptin and tell your brain that you're starving. MiRNA from the numerous fat cells bring the same message to most of the body in the form of episomes. Remember, 70 percent of your resting metabolism is from the liver, brain, and kidneys. When the metabolism of these organs drops, no amount of exercise can overcome that. More exercise makes a patient with chronic obesity more hungry.

The only way to fight this is with diet medications. Find a physician certified by the American Board of Obesity Medicine who has a good bioelectric impedance weight scale so that you can track your muscle mass. It will be discouraging to see the 5 to 10 percent loss of muscle mass as you lose weight, but it's more important to lose as much weight as possible in the first six to nine months. Then, at the plateau, start the low-weight, high-repetition (twenty-five reps, three sets, four times a week) exercises on a high-protein diet (2.4 mg/d protein per kg of lean body weight). With more exercise comes more hunger, so you'll need diet medications more than ever.

November 6, 2015—I had 44.2 pounds of muscle, as measured by a bioelectric impedance scale, with 235.1 pounds of weight.

June 23, 2015—I began going to the Stormont Obesity Clinic run by Dr. Jennifer Scheid, who is board certified in obesity medicine. After a month of weight lifting and water aerobics, I weighed 244.8 pounds with 46.1 pounds of muscle mass.

May 23, 2017—After diet medications, continuing an Atkins-type diet, and walking only one to two miles per day, I returned home from a wedding weekend in Philadelphia and a National Lipid Association meeting. I weighed 199 pounds with 37.4 pounds of muscle mass.

My present goal is to do twenty-five repetitions of low weights each day, alternating between my legs and upper body, trying especially to gain muscle in my legs. I will also try to eat 2.4 grams of protein/kg of lean body weight, which is about a gram of protein per pound of lean body weight.

Lean body weight at 199 pounds is 150 pounds. My visceral fat is 13; normal is 9 or less. I hope to reach my visceral fat goal of 9 or less with more muscle mass. That's more important than the actual total pounds of weight.

If I can get my waist under 40 inches and my visceral fat to 9, I hope to increase my adiponectin, which will improve my insulin resistance. My insulin level is 8.4, which is normal. However, I have type 2 diabetes, which means that enough of the beta cells in my pancreas have died so that I can't increase my insulin to a level normally seen in insulin resistance.

I will report my future efforts on my blog at http://meandgin.blogspot.com/.

Summary: Multiple diet medications have helped me maintain my weight loss from 280 to 200 pounds since February 2006. I think that Atkins has been essential, because I eat ad libitum and *I'm never hungry*. Although I didn't really *lose* weight on Atkins, I stopped *gaining* weight, even though I decreased my exercise from two hours per day to walking twenty to forty minutes per day. Also I lost significant weight when I added the diet medications. On January 1, 2018, I weighed 204.2 pounds.

Glossary

Blood Test Terms

LDL-C: The *C* stands for cholesterol. This is the bad cholesterol, which is determined from a blood test. It's a calculated number and is often discordant with the newer, better LDL-P test.

LDL-P: The number of particles (P) that carry the cholesterol is the best predictor of cardiovascular risk. It's determined by a blood test and an NMR machine. ApoB is another way to measure atherogenic particles. High-fat diets make large LDL-P, whereas low-fat diets make for more small, dense LDL-P. There is much confusion about the importance of size relative to risk stratification. The National Lipid Association meetings preach that size doesn't matter most of the time (no double entendre intended).

HDL-C: This has been called the good cholesterol. Ratios are often used to determine cardiovascular risk. The AIM-HIGH trial and the fact that there are pro-inflammatory or bad HDL-Cs makes the ratio with HDL-C less reliable. Low-fat diets lower HDL-C, and high-fat diets raise HDL-C.

HDL-P: The particle number will rise with the HDL-C to approximately 60 dl/ml. At this point, as the HDL-C goes higher, the size of the HDL-P gets larger. What does it all mean? It's a conundrum, because the critical test is the functionality of the HDL-P. There is no clinical lab test for functionality at this time.

Triglycerides: Three fatty acids make up a triglyceride. Low-carbohydrate diets have low triglycerides, and low-fat diets have high triglycerides.

Tubby Factor: I coined this term because the technical term *non-HDL cholesterol* was too confusing. This is the second-best predictor of cardiovascular risk. It is all the cholesterol without the HDLc. Take the total cholesterol level on the lipid panel and subtract the HDLc. This is also often discordant with the LDLc, especially in people with metabolic syndrome.

Medical Imaging Terms

CAC (coronary calcium score): This is a CT scan of the heart that can show if patients have plaque in their coronary arteries. No IV or dye is involved.

CIMT (carotid intima medial wall thickness): An ultrasound of the carotid arteries in the neck measures the thickness of the wall of the carotid. This is different from the duplex carotid ultrasound that measures the flow of the blood in the carotid and determines how much blockage is in the carotid.

Diabetic Terms

Metabolic Syndrome: This is a prediabetic state that combines apple obesity, high blood pressure, high triglycerides, and low HDLc. TG/HDLc ratio should be less than 3.

Hgb A1C: Hemoglobin A1C is a blood test to determine the average glucose level in the blood over the previous one or two months.

Prediabetes: A fasting glucose of 100 or greater.

Apple Obesity: A waist larger than 40 inches in men or 35 inches in women; smaller for Asians.

High Blood Pressure: Greater than 130 systolic. My preference is to get it between 90 and 120, or until you feel dizzy or light-headed.

High Triglycerides: Greater than 150. My preference is to get nonfasting TG under 100 with niacin and Lovaza (fish oil).

Low HDL-C: Below 40 for men and 50 for women.

Anabolic: Using energy to build body substances.

Catabolic: Breaking down substances to make energy.

Reduced Obese: A reduced-obese person has lost a significant amount of weight and now has a metabolism different from that of obese people and normal-weight people. The body of a reduced obese uses several compensatory mechanisms to gain weight.

Set Point: "Obesity is a consequence of the complex interplay between genetics and environment. Several studies have shown that body weight is maintained at a stable range, known as the 'set-point,' despite the variability in energy intake and expenditure. Additionally, it has been shown that the body is more efficient protecting against weight loss during caloric deprivation compared to conditions of weight gain with overfeeding, suggesting an adaptive role of protection during periods of low food intake. Emerging evidence on bariatric surgery outcomes, particularly gastric bypass, suggests a novel role of these surgical procedures in establishing a new set-point by alterations in body weight regulatory physiology, therefore resulting in sustainable weight loss results. Continuing research is necessary to elucidate the biological mechanisms responsible for this change, which may offer new options for the global burden of obesity." (Farias, M. M., Cuevas, A. M., Rodriguez, F. (2011). "Set-point Theory and Obesity." *Metabolic Syndrome & Related Disorders, 9*(2), 85–89. doi:10.1089/met.2010.0090)

Plateau: After an 8 percent weight loss, it becomes difficult to lose additional weight. This plateau is usually reached after six to nine months of strict dieting.

Resettlement Point: Is this a new term for plateau? Obese people have high levels of leptin. Some believe this is a resistance as with insulin, whereas others believe the obese have a high leptin threshold. Fat cells make leptin, but as fat cells shrink, less leptin is made. If the threshold is high in the obese and the leptin level drops below a threshold that alerts the brain that the body is starving, the body starts compensatory mechanisms to regain weight.

Energy Gap: "These formulas would predict an energy gap of 190–200 kcal/day for a 100 kg person losing 10% of body weight and an energy gap of 280–300 kcal/day for this same person losing 15% of body weight ... The energy gap for weight loss maintenance can provide an estimate of how much behavior change is required to maintain a given amount of weight loss. This analysis indicates that in order to create and maintain significant body weight loss (i.e. obesity treatment) large behavioral changes are needed. This is in stark contrast to primary obesity prevention in which small behavioral changes can eliminate the small energy imbalance that occurs before the body has gained significant weight. Because the body has not previously stored this 'new' excess energy, it does not defend against the behavioral strategies as happens when the body loses weight." (Hill, J. O., Peters, J. C., & Wyatt, H. R. (2009)."Using the Energy Gap to Address Obesity: A Commentary." *Journal of the Academy of Nutrition and Dietetics 109*(11), 1848–1853. doi:10.1016/j.jada.2009.08.007)

Leptin Threshold: "Dieting means less fat in your body's fat cells, and it also means a lower level of leptin. When you go below your personal leptin threshold, your brain thinks you're starving. The body has ways of handling this apparent crisis, initiating a number of processes designed to keep you from starving, and raise the level of leptin back up above your personal leptin threshold. Unfortunately these processes can also sabotage your diet." (Smith, Jody. "The Hormone Leptin Affects Weight Loss and Weight Gain." *Women's Health & Wellness.* http://www.webmd.com/diet/features/the-facts-on-leptin-faq?ecd=wnl_day_060310)

Leptin Resistance: "Although leptin is a circulating signal that reduces appetite, obese individuals generally exhibit an unusually high circulating concentration of leptin. These people are said to be resistant to the effects of leptin, in much the same way that people with type 2 diabetes are resistant to the effects of insulin. The high sustained concentrations of leptin from the enlarged adipose stores result in leptin desensitization. The pathway of leptin control in obese people might be flawed at some point so the body does not adequately receive the satiety feeling subsequent to eating." (Taken from "Leptin" at Wikipedia.com.)

Sponge Syndrome: I coined this term because the definitions above are complicated and not yet fully understood. After losing eighty pounds, I regained fifty-eight pounds, despite two to three hours of exercise a day, over a forty-three-month period. At an average of 1.35 pounds per month, I regained weight like a sponge. My body's energy gap, which develops during weight loss, had gradually increased as I initially lost weight. A very obese person can have 80 billion fat cells that don't go away when they lose a hundred pounds, and shrunken fat cells don't generate much leptin. A low leptin level tells the brain that the body is starving, while all those billions of shrunken fat cells act like a sponge for any increase in calories.

Moral Hazard of Obesity: When someone becomes obese, there's a general belief that it's their own fault and that they should lose weight only through deprivation and exercise. The idea that weight loss can be maintained with a high-fat diet and little exercise seems impossible to most people. Thus people have been slow to accept Atkins and low-carbohydrate, high-fat diets, as well as the idea that you can't outrun your fork. Morally it doesn't seem right to people who are naturally thin.

National Weight Control Registry: The NWCR found that people who maintained weight loss did achieve some aspects of success. Many guidelines base their recommendations on NWCR research findings.

1. They weighed themselves every day. If they gained three to five pounds, they had a plan for what to do about it immediately.
2. They tended to have little variety in their food.
3. They splurged less on food over holidays.
4. They ate 1,385 calories per day, though the facilitator said they were underreporting.
5. They ate 4.87 meals each day.
6. They linked behaviors to something more than just losing weight. For example, they used walking as their social time. They linked good behaviors to something they wanted to do.
7. They often had recently experienced a life-changing event, such as divorce or a new job.
8. They walked about five miles a day or engaged in equivalent exercise.

"The National Weight Control Registry documented the metabolic and behavioral cost of maintaining a weight loss for more than 5 years. The average weight loss was 30 kg (66 lbs) and minimum maintenance 13.6 kg (29.92 lbs). The results are instructive. Both men and women consumed a low-fat diet (24%) and exercised to use 470 and 360 kcal/d, respectively. The net energy balance was 918 kcal/day for women and 1225 kcal/d for men. These reduced obese ate an average of five meals a day and conducted a very regimented existence." (Dubnov-Raz, G., & Berry, E. (1995). "The Dietary Treatment of Obesity." *Medical Clinics of North America*, *95*(5), 939–952. This quotation comes from page 945.)

Ancel Keys and the Great Starvation Experiment: Compare this World War II experiment to the eight NWCR items listed above. Thirty-two volunteers were fed approximately 1,550 calories per day for six months, walked three miles a day, and suffered mentally and physically. When a few of them who hadn't lost weight were caught eating garbage, they were kicked out of the experiment. This is the same insane diet to which most guidelines tell patients to adhere today.

The good news is that we now have drugs that can prevent the severe hunger. The bad news is that most physicians and patients either don't know about them or don't want to take a diet medication for the rest of their lives.

Obesity Drugs

1. Orlistat—Orlistat inhibits gastric and pancreatic that help digest fat. Impairing fat absorption leads to weight loss. "Interestingly, orlistat can reverse liver steatosis but not adipocyte hypertrophy." I do not recommend this drug; it comes with the risk of too many hygiene accidents.

2. Phentermine—Phentermine is a sympathomimetic amine. It is a scheduled DEA drug and label directions allow them to be taken for only one year. It's good to add to Belviq for a combination similar to Phen/Fen, which was taken off the market.

3. Belviq (lorcaserin)—Similar to fenfuramate (Pondimin), this is a 5-HT 2c receptor agonist (5-HT: 5-hydroxytryptamine), though more specific than Pondimin. Fifty percent of people respond to this drug. After two months, if you've had only a poor response, add low-dose phentermine (off-label). Physicians need a DEA number to prescribe this.

4. Contrave (naltrexone and bupropion)—The new trend is to use two drugs in combination to get better results, since the brain can outsmart a single drug in six to twelve months. Naltrexone is an antagonist of opioid receptors in pro-opiomelanocortin (POMCs) neurons. Bupropion is a noradrenaline and dopamine reuptake inhibitor. Adding amylin (a peptide coreleased with insulin by pancreatic B cells) to these drugs seems to result in better outcomes, because of the modulation of the melanocortin (MC) pathway (increasing the expression of MC4 receptor in hypothalamic neurons). Again we see that a combination of drugs—in this case, three off-label drugs—gets better results.

5. Topiramate—Your physician does not need a DEA number to prescribe this, but you shouldn't take it if you can't take narcotic medications. Topiramate is an antiepileptic drug that acts as antagonist of AMPA (a-amino-3-hydroxy-5-methyl-4-isoxazolepropionic acid) receptors and positively modulates γ-aminobutyric acid (GABA) receptors. This drug is associated with memory loss.

6. Liraglutide—Liraglutide is a glucagon-like peptide 1 receptor agonist (GLP-1RA), first approved as an antidiabetic drug and, more recently, in higher doses as an anti-obesity drug. GLP-1 is an endogenous incretin secreted by L cells in the distal intestine.

   (a) Liraglutide increases GLP-1 levels, reduces food ingestion and appetite, and modifies food preferences, namely, improving eating and decreasing emotional eating, which increases weight loss.

   (b) GLP-1 was described as having anti-adipogenic, anti-lipogenic, and prolipolytic effects in human mature adipocytes.

   (c) GLP-1R is more expressed in adipocytes from VAT of obese T2DM patients, compared with lean patients. Liraglutide can improve insulin sensitivity, even in insulin-resistant models.

   (d) Liraglutide slows gastric emptying, which helps to reduce food intake.

(e) Liraglutide activates GLP-1R in the central nervous system, leading to an increase in BAT activity and energy expenditure.

(f) Liraglutide increases Omentin, an adipokine mainly produced by VAT; levels are decreased in T2DM. Increases glucose transport induced by insulin, hence improving insulin sensitivity and glucose metabolism, which could contribute to improving insulin action.

When I wanted to lose another 5 percent of my weight because my clinic incorrectly told me I needed to in order to stay on my diet medications, I increased my Victoza to 3.0 mg a day for a month. I suffered no side effects and it worked.

CHAPTER 23

How I Got Fired by My Endocrinologist

On December 21, 2017, during the Christmas holidays, I had a fasting glucose of 240 when I reported my levels. I was surprised that my endocrinologist gave me a pass. Four months later, right after cataract surgery after fasting but getting IV Ringer's Lactate and then a small muffin post-op, my glucose was 248 and my insulin level was 8.4.

My endocrinologist immediately wanted me to add a sulfonylurea such as glipizide. I told her that when I was practicing, I got away from sulfonylureas because they eventually milk the liver dry of insulin and the patient has to go on insulin injections. She agreed that was true. I said I would be willing to go on Actos (Pioglitazone) at a low dose, since that seems to be the best drug for insulin resistance. She doesn't like Actos because it has been associated with osteoporosis, and I already have osteopenia. I remember being surprised to find that I have osteopenia, because I've always been heavy and lifted weights over the years. However, I had been on Actos.

A few years ago, I had gone to lunch with Dr. Eric Westman and he had suggested that I stop Actos to help my weight loss on Atkins. When I did, I quickly lost ten pounds, but my fasting glucose shot up to 300!

I told my endocrinologist that, of course, that weight loss was just water, which is probably why you have to be careful giving it to borderline heart failure patients. She disagreed and insisted that it was lipid weight. I'm not sure what that means and I was pretty sure she was wrong, but I moved on.

We agreed that I would do three- or four-hour post-prandial glucose. If I was running greater than 180, we would start Actos. I thought that we had reached a good compromise.

I asked if we should get another DEXA scan, since it had been three years. She said she wasn't certain that Medicare would pay for it. I told her that if she wrote that she wanted to make certain I didn't develop osteoporosis by stopping testosterone IM, the DEXA scan would be approved, but she wanted to look that up.

She agreed with me that getting insulin levels with fasting glucose to pick up insulin resistance early in people with FBG of less than 100 is a good idea. Then I asked if I could have an insulin level with my next fasting glucose. She said no. I said I had an insulin level of 8.4 with a glucose of 248 after fasting and IV Ringer's lactate for my cataract surgery. She said I had DM2 and didn't need an insulin level. I said that if I took Actos, I wanted to know if my insulin level would get lower with better glucose control.

I said my HDLc/triglyceride ratio was less than 3. My *non*-fasting TG was 99.

My systolic BP was 116 on ramipril for DM2 and Diltazem for atrial fibrillation. My waist was 41.5 inches, and I wanted to try to get it under 40 inches. My bioelectrical impedance scale said my visceral fat was 14.

When I did my lipscience advanced lipid study by NMR, my IR score was in the middle, in the 40s—not a strong score for IR, even though my VLDL was a little high because it was nonfasting.

I knew I was DM2, I knew I was IR even though my insulin level was normal.

I thought I had lost enough beta cells in the pancreas that I couldn't muster a high insulin level like a younger person with IR would have. DM1 may have a zero insulin level. I didn't want to get there. I hoped that by losing more visceral fat, I could increase my adiponectin to help my IR.

I told my endocrinologist I was in Asia and Hawaii from January 11 to March 18, and I was running in the high 170s FBS even though I was walking at least 10,000 steps a day. When I came home, my Hgb A1c was 7.7. I tried to stay on Atkins, but on vacation I was probably not in nutritional ketosis. I was not taking my serum ketone levels, so I can't know for certain.

I had been in Topeka for a month and had had fasting serum ketone greater than 0.4 every day except for 0.2 and 0.4 on two separate mornings. My fasting glucose had been in the 140s.

Thus I told my endocrinologist I thought my Hgb. A1c was back at 6.5.

We compromised and agreed I would start doing post-prandial glucoses as I mentioned above but no insulin levels.

I told her I knew I was maintaining my low-carb diet because I had been in serum nutritional ketosis each morning in the last month. She was surprised there was a serum finger stick home test for ketones and didn't know anything about it. This was a young endocrinologist who had gotten out of training a year earlier.

She wanted to fire me because she thought my questions indicated that I didn't trust her. When I told her that I liked and trusted her, and that I wanted her to continue as my doctor, she relented. When I got home, however, her nurse called and said she had transferred me to another physician.

Here's the post-prandial glucose as requested by my endocrinologist:
April 23, 2018: Two and a half hours after three tacos for lunch—166 glucose.
April 24, 2018: Three hours after three eggs and three slices of bacon for breakfast—149 glucose. Four hours after Mexican lamb soup and a premium clear protein drink (20g protein, no carbs for lunch)—145 glucose.

Thus on a strict low-carbohydrate diet, I am good on my post-prandial glucose and so far I don't need Actos. My morning ketone level on April 25 was 1.1.

I would still like to get a couple of insulin levels with fasting glucose. I hope my next endocrinologist will allow it.

Index

Printed in the United States
By Bookmasters